Stop the Depression Crisis

Navya

CHAPTER I

INTRODUCTION

Depression is a serious and pervasive common mental disorder (CMD) with a striking

global presence; the condition had a point prevalence of 4.7% worldwide in 2010 (Ferrari et al.,

2013), meaning over 303 million people struggled with this condition over the period of

just1year. Persons with depression can experience reduced quality of life and significant

impairment across a number of domains, including physical, social, cognitive and parental

functioning (Cotrena, Branco, Shansis, & Fonseca, 2016; Löwe et al., 2008; Cuijpers, Weitz,

Karyotaki, Garber, & Andersson, 2015).

The condition is also burdensome to an individual's physical health, with depressive

disorders alone accounting for 65.5 million disability-adjusted life years (DALYs) worldwide

(WHO, 2008). Nearly 85% of those DALYs are accounted for by those living with depression in

low- and middle-income countries (WHO, 2008). The brutal impact of this mental health

condition is expected to only intensify, advancing from the position of the fourth-leading cause

of global disease burden in 1990 to an anticipated second place in 2020 (Murray, Lopez &

WHO, 1996).

Depression is a condition that disproportionately burdens women, who are nearly twice

(OR 1.95) as likely to suffer from the condition than men (Salk, Hyde, & Abramson, 2017).

These odds are further complicated by the hormonal fluctuations that develop as a result of

pregnancy and childbirth (Altemus, Sarvaiya, & Epperson, 2014; Wisner et al., 2013; Stewart,

Robertson, Dennis, Grace, & Wallington, 2003; Gavin et al., 2005) and the often difficult role transitions women experience as a result of these life events (Epifanio, Genna, De Luca, Roccella & La Grutta, 2015; Ngai & Ngu, 2015).

Though the majority of the current literature on postpartum depression (PPD) is based on populations from high-income countries (Maselko, 2017), the extant literature indicates that the incidence of PPD is greater among women in low- and middle-income countries (Villegas, McKay, Dennis & Ross, 2011; Fisher et al., 2012; Parsons, Young, Rochat, Kringelback & Stein, 2012; WHO, 2008;), and the physical and mental health consequences of the condition on both mother and child are much more dire in these settings (Gelaye, Rondon,Araya, & Williams, 2016; Nachega et al., 2012).

While maternal mental health has been extensively linked to poorer child outcomes such as undernutrition and stunting, explanation of the underlying mechanisms responsible for this link are underrepresented. In a recent review of the extant literature on maternal depression and child health outcomes, Surkan and colleagues (Surkan, Kennedy, Hurley, & Black, 2011) found a significant association between maternal depression and early childhood stunting and underweight. The authors emphasized that the reasons for this association remain unclear. They consequently issued a charge to the greater public and global health communities to identify the mechanisms at work leading to the children of mothers with depression to a predisposition to poorer health. To emphasize the crucial impact identification of these mechanisms would have, Surkan and colleagues calculated that the elimination of maternal depressive symptoms worldwide would lead to 23 to 29% fewer children who are underweight and stunted.

The current study addresses the gap in the literature Surkan et al. (2011) have identified through the lens of maternal behavior. Though numerous studies evidence a specific roster of maternal behaviors known to affect child health, there is presently no literature identifying the differential rates of these behaviors demonstrated in mothers with depression and mothers without the condition at baseline. Additionally, though social support and women's empowerment and autonomy both have identified and pronounced relationships with depression, it is currently unclear how these two constructs may function within the relationship between maternal depression and child health outcomes.

The primary aim of the current study is therefore to investigate in a sample of Ugandan mothers of children 0 to 23 months how maternal behaviors promoting child health differ in the presence or absence of postpartum depression and to explore how perceived social support and women's empowerment and autonomy may moderate the relationship between PPD and the adoption of these health-promoting behaviors. The study is based on cross-sectional, baseline data collected for a project sponsored by the Food for the Hungry, an international relief and development organization in Uganda, and in partnership with the Global Mental Health Lab at Teachers College, Columbia University and World Vision, International. The study's sample is taken from mothers residing in Northern Uganda, a region deeply afflicted both by depression (1486.4 to 1630 years lived with disability per 100,000 years; Ferrari et al., 2013) and poor maternal health and child health outcomes (Singla, Kumbakumba, & Aboud, 2015).

The current study offers crucial insight into the impact of maternal depression on maternal behavior, and consequently, child health. Identification of the specific behaviors differentially impacted by the presence or absence of PPD would offer streamlined, concrete recommendations for developing targeted yet comprehensive evidence-based programs that address the practices most significantly impacting child health.

CHAPTER II

LITERATURE REVIEW

Depression in the Perinatal Period

Maternal depression is a comprehensive term covering a range of depressive conditions affecting peripartum women. Subsumed under this term are postpartum psychosis, antenatal (or prenatal) depression, and postpartum (or postnatal) depression (PPD; Shidhaye & Giri, 2014). Prominent symptoms include crying more than usual, anger, withdrawal from loved ones, feeling distant from one's baby, excess worry or anxiousness, thoughts of self-harm or harm to one's child, and self-doubt around parenting ability (Centers for Disease Control and Prevention [CDC], 2018, para. 6). Perinatally, the condition is associated with increased obstetric complications such as increased risk of preeclampsia gestational hypertension, and greater likelihood of need for operative deliveries and epidural anesthesia (Bonari et al., 2004; Chung, Lau, Yip, Chiu & Lee, 2001).

Additionally, the conditions maternal depression subsumes compound upon one another; antenatal depression is reliably identified as a significant predictor of PPD (Garman, Schneider & Lnd, 2019; Ngai & Ngu, 2015; Roomruangwong, Kanchanatawan, Sirivichayakul, & Maes, 2016; Underwood, Waldie, D'Souza, Peterson, & Morton, 2016), the repercussions for which are manifold for both mother and child. PPD has been identified as a predictor of poorer mother-infant bonding and infant emotional and behavioral development at 1 year and poorer child psychological functioning at up to 10 years (Choi et al., 2017; Verkuijl et al., 2014). The infants of mothers with depression also face adverse health outcomes such as low gestational age at birth, low birthweight, increased likelihood of preterm birth and greater likelihood of requiring

neonatal intensive care unit (NICU) admission (Chung et al., 2001; Grigoriadis et al., 2013; Suri

et al., 2007). While child outcomes for this condition are well-researched, its impact on maternal

health remains severely understudied. The extant literature does identify a particular

susceptibility of those with this condition to postpartum fatigue and a reduced capacity for self-

care (Khatun et al., 2018).

The Global Burden of Postpartum Depression

Although a global prevalence rate for PPD has not yet been identified, rates between 1%

and 20% are most commonly cited in Western countries (Gaynes et al., 2005; Gavin et al., 2005;

Woody, Ferrari, Siskind, Whiteford, & Harris; 2017). Upon examining the prevalence of PPD

by region, however, estimates vary substantially both within and across areas. The United States

identifies rates similar to the aforementioned estimate, ranging from 9 to 17% (McCue Horwitz,

Briggs-Gowan, Storfer-Isser, & Carter, 2007; Vesga-Lopez et al., 2008). Rates within other high-

income countries such as Australia (16%; Woolhouse, 2014) France, and Portugal (15.6% and

14.6%, respectively; Gorman et al., 2004) are also consistent with this range. Studies done in

Southern European countries indicate a prevalence range of PPD between 4.4% and 22.8%

(Escriba-Aguir & Artazcoz, 2011; Lambrinoudaki, Rizos, Armeni, et al., 2010) found in Spain

and Greece, respectively. Northern Europe saw a range of 10.1% to 16.5% in Norway and

Sweden, respectively (Glavin, Smith, & Sørum, 2009; Kerstis, Engström, Sundquist, et al.,

2012). PPD in the Central European countries of the Netherlands and Germany had a range of

8.5% to 22%, respectively (Meijer, Beijers, van Pampus, et al., 2014; Zaers, Waschke, & Ehlert,

2008). In Poland , PPD had a prevalence of 16% (Dudek, Jaeschke, Siwek, et al. 2014). A cohort

study done in Belgium, Germany, Italy, Poland, and Spain saw a 11.0% PPD prevalence (Grote,

Vik, von Kries, et al., 2010)

Within less developed regions of the world, the variance of prevalence rates tends to be

greater. This is perhaps truest for populations in Asia. With numerous studies on maternal

depression covering this region, estimates are reportedly as low as 4.9%, as in Nepal (Dørheim

Ho-Yen, Tschudi Bondevik, Eberhard-Gran, & Bjorvatn, 2007), and as high as 33%, as in

Vietnam (Fisher, Morrow, Ngoc, & Anh, 2004). Rates in China fall at the more moderate level

of this range, with reports ranging from 9.4% (Wu et al., 2014) to 27.4% (Deng, Xiong, Jiang,

Luo & Chen, 2014). Countries in the Middle East are also quite varied. Al Hinai & Al Hinai

(2014) found a 13.5% prevalence rate for postnatal depression among postpartum mothers in

Oman, while Husain et al. (2006) found a rate nearly triple that amount (36%) in Pakistan for the

same disorder.

Finally, in Africa, rates of maternal depression are consistently elevated compared to

other regions of the world. Chibanda et al. (2010) found in a Zimbabwean population with a high

HIV-prevalence a rate of about 33% for maternal depression. Studies among South African

populations found a prevalence of PPD in the range of 34.7% to 50.3% (Tomlinson et al., 2006;

Stellenberg & Abrahams, 2015).

Maternal Depression in LMICs

A recent systematic review of the extant literature on common perinatal mental disorders

(CPMDs) found that one in five postpartum women in LMICs experience a CPMD (Fisher et al.,

2012), estimates that far exceed the reported rates in high-income settings of 13% for postpartum depression(Hendrick, Altshiler, Cohen, & Stowe, 1998; O'hara & Swain, 1996). The review identifies a number of risk factors associated with having one of these disorders, but the factors presenting the greatest risk include low socioeconomic status (upper limit of OR range=13.2), low empathy or support from one's intimate partner (9.4), unintended pregnancy (8.8), intimate partner violence (IPV; 6.75), and insufficient social support (6.1; Fisher et al., 2012).

A recent systematic review and meta-analysis corroborates the experience of IPV as a risk-factor for probable PPD. The review found that women who endorsed having experienced IPV during pregnancy were three times as likely (OR=3.1) to have PPD than those who did not (Howard, Oram, Galley, Trevillion & Feder, 2013).

Studies included in reviews by Sawyer, Ayers, and Smith (2010) and Wittkowski, Gardner, Bunton, and Edge (2014) support Fisher et al. (2012)'s findings, emphasizing the impact of low social support and a poor relationship with one's intimate partner on the incidence of PPD across a variety of African countries. However, both reviews did not find low socioeconomic status to be a significant risk factor for PPD.

Prevalence of Depression in Uganda

Reported prevalence rates for depressive disorders in Uganda have varied considerably across studies in the last 15 years, since research on the condition has become more frequent. Estimates have been as low as 6.1% (Nakku, Nakasi, & Mirembe, 2006) and as high as 61.3% (Fischer, Ramaswamy, Fischer-Flores & Mugisha, 2018). This wide variance may be attributable to a number of factors, including the evaluation of specific sub-populations like HIV-infected individuals, internally displaced persons, pregnant or postpartum women, or people residing in specific post-conflict regions of Uganda. It is worth noting, however, that significant variance is found within the categories of these studies as well; this may be a result of the different instruments used in these studies to measure depression and their validity for use in the population. The reported prevalence rates and conditions for these studies are explored below.

Depression has been most readily explored in Uganda in the context of HIV/AIDS. Even within this subset of the Ugandan population, the distribution of prevalence rates for probable depression is wide, with some estimates falling as low as 9-10% (Wagner et al., 2014; Mwesiga et al., 2015) and others as high as 64% (Stangl et al., 2007). According to findings from Nakasujja et al., (2010), HIV-infected individuals were nearly three times (OR=2.86) more likely to be depressed than their uninfected counterparts. Reports with higher reported rates may be partially explained by frequent reporting of neurovegetative symptoms such as poor appetite, fatigue, weight loss and insomnia, symptoms often associated with HIV/AIDS. Indeed, Wagner, Holloway, Ghosh-Dastidar, Kityo, and Mugyenyi (2011) found that trouble sleeping (17%), fatigue (18%) and poor appetite (23%) were their most reported symptoms apart from depressed mood (19%), findings corroborated by results from other studies (Psaros et al., 2015). To account for this, some studies utilized modified scales for depression either excluding somatic symptoms or placing greater weight on cognitive symptoms (Kaharuza et al., 2006; Wagner et al., 2011). Findings from these scales still indicated a greater prevalence of depression among individuals infected with HIV. These findings are particularly meaningful for women, whom the authors found were more likely to be infected with HIV than men in the sample. (Kaharuza et al., 2006; Wagner et al., 2011).

8

Within the general Ugandan population, point prevalence rates for depression hover between 9 and 29% (Kaida et al., 2014; Kinyanda et al., 2011; Ovuga, Boardman, & Wasserman, 2005). In a study including samples from 2 districts in Uganda, one with greater conflict exposure and one with considerably less, a significant difference in prevalence was found in favor of the conflict exposed district (26.3% prevalence in Adjumani district compared to 6% in Bugiri district; Ovuga et al., 2005). One study implemented around the same time identified prevalence rates more than twice this estimate among internally displaced persons residing in post-conflict Northern Uganda (67.4% prevalence; Roberts, Ocaka, Browne, Oyok, & Sondorp, 2008).

Considering the extant body of literature on the prevalence of depression in Uganda, reported estimates tend to hover in a range much greater than the estimated global prevalence of 4.7% for the disorder (Ferrari et al., 2013). The Ugandan population's exposure to a number of factors increasing risk for the condition—including HIV infection, conflict exposure, internal displacement, poverty and food insecurity—emphasizes the need for greater attention to the treatment, policy, and consequences of depression.

Prevalence of Depression among Women in Uganda

Consistent with reports from global and western depression prevalence studies, women are twice as likely to have depression than men in Uganda (Kinyanda, Hoskins, Nakku, Nawaz, & Patel, 2011), a gender gap which widens in the context of HIV infection. Tsai et al. (2012) found in a sample of men and women enrolled for HIV treatment in rural Uganda that women were more than five times as likely to meet criteria for probable depression. Similar odds were found in a study of internally displaced men and women from districts in Northern Uganda, which found that women were over four times as likely to demonstrate depressive symptomatology as men ([OR=4.32]; Roberts et al., 2008). Kinyanda, Hoskins et al. (2011) offer some insight into the differential impact of depression on men and women, reporting that the association between female gender and depression is greatly mediated by a greater incidence of negative life events and higher stress scores among women. Additionally, Cooper-Vince et al. (2018) observed in a hotspot analysis of the geospatial clustering of depression in rural Uganda that areas with greater water insecurity increased risk for depressive symptoms among women only, which they ascribed to stress induced from the primary role women play in the obtainment and use of water for household tasks like cooking, cleaning and childcare.

An additional role unique to women that may impact the risk for mental illness is pregnancy. While there is a paucity of literature evaluating depression prevalence in pregnant and postpartum women compared to matched, non-pregnant controls in LMICs, community-based studies in Turkey do shed some light on this comparison. The comparison of pregnant women to non-pregnant matched controls in Turkey found no statistically significant differences between the two groups, though it did find that the factors associated with a participant's score on the Beck Depression Inventory (BDI) differed by pregnancy status (Caliskan, Oncu, Kose, Ocaktan, & Ozdemir, 2007). The researchers found that age, spouse's educational level, family income, and the number of people living in her home were predictive of depression score for pregnant women while mental health history and negative life events predicted depression among non-pregnant women (Caliskan, Oncu, Kose, Ocaktan, & Ozdemir, 2007).

In contrast to these findings in Turkey, Fatoye, Adeyemi, and Oladimeji (2004) found in a cross-sectional comparison of depression and anxiety symptoms among third-trimester pregnant women and non-pregnant matched controls that pregnant women demonstrated both disorders at significantly higher levels than non-pregnant women. Further still, the sociodemographic characteristics such as age, education level, socioeconomic status and parity Caliskan and colleagues (2007) found to be predictive of depression among pregnant women were not associated with either depression or anxiety severity among the pregnant women in this Nigerian sample. The researchers did find positive correlations between depression and participation in a polygamous family structure, previous delivery difficulties, ever having had an abortion, and puerperal complication or illness (Fatoye, Adeyemi, & Oladimeji, 2004). It is important to note the differential recruiting methods and inclusion criteria for these two studies, however, as they may contribute to the difference in findings. While Caliskan and colleagues (2007) recruited all participants, pregnant women and matched controls, from a single primary health care center, Fatoye et al. (2004) recruited their pregnant participants from the antenatal clinic of a hospital and their non-pregnant controls from a family planning clinic in the same hospital. The recruitment methods of the latter study may have accommodated some bias with regard to reproductive values between the two groups.

Additionally, Fatoye and colleagues (2004) set no apparent limits on matched-control participants for pregnancy history while criteria for the controls in Caliskan et al. (2007)'s study required that they had given birth at least1year prior to study participation, meaning no nulliparous women were included in this study. Finally, Fatoye and colleagues focused their study on third-trimester pregnant women, or women whose gestation was 36 weeks or greater, while Caliskan and colleagues recruited women in all stages of pregnancy, though no statistically significant difference was found across women in different trimesters of pregnancy in this study (Caliskan et al., 2007).

The disproportionate impact of depression on women only intensifies at the intersection of pregnancy and HIV infection, as indicated by the findings of a cross-sectional validation study for the Center for Epidemiologic Studies Depression (CES-D) scale among HIV-infected and uninfected pregnant women in northern Uganda (Natamba et al., 2014). In this study, the prevalence rate among HIV-infected women (52.9%) was nearly double that of their uninfected counterparts (28.7%). This finding is contested, however, by Kaida et al. (2014), who longitudinally compared depression severity in a sample of HIV-infected Ugandan women across their non-pregnant, pregnant and postpartum periods. The authors found no difference in depression symptom severity across these pregnancy statuses, suggesting that HIV infection may make a more impactful contribution to depression severity than pregnancy. As a result of exposure to compounding life stressors like HIV infection, which demonstrates a greater prevalence among women in Uganda (WHO, 2010; Ugandan Ministry of Health, 2012), puerperal women in Uganda are particularly vulnerable to depressive symptoms.

Risk and Protective Factors for Maternal Depression in Uganda

As is the case for most LMICs, mothers in Uganda demonstrate an elevated risk for PPD than their counterparts in developed countries. While poverty and economic stress are identified as common risk factors for maternal depression across LMICs, the additional risk factors for this condition appear to vary geographically. Parsons et al. (2012) highlight the birth of a female child when a male was preferred as a reported contributor to the onset of PPD in India while in Sub-Saharan Africa (SSA), the relationships between depression and marital conflict as well as lack of support are more pronounced (Sawyer, Ayers & Smith, 2010). Women in northern Uganda, where the current study takes place, may face even greater vulnerability to depression due to their more frequent experience of adverse life events, often related to the armed conflict in this area, and the high prevalence of HIV/AIDS (Mugisha, Muyinda, Malamba & Kinyanda, 2015).

Sociodemographic factors. The literature on the sociodemographic risk and protective factors specific to this population will be explored below. Its organization is informed by the conceptual framework adopted by the WHO Commission on Social Determinants of Health (Solar & Irwin, 2010) and the systematic review of the prevalence and determinants of non-psychotic perinatal mental disorders in LMICs conducted by Fisher and colleagues (2012).*Age.* Merely two studies were found in the current literature review reporting significant findings for the association of age and maternal depression in Uganda. Findings from Nakku et al. (2006) showed that young age (age 10-19) increased the risk for major depression at six weeks postpartum (OR=3.49). Conversely, Natamba et al. (2017) found older maternal age to be significantly associated with depressive symptoms, as measured by participant score on the CES-D.

Broadening the context to major depression among the general population in Uganda, Kinyanda, Woodburn et al. (2011) found older age to be independently associated with probably major depression within a sample of men and women from 14 districts in Uganda, noting that the condition's prevalence increased with each age category above 35 years. Among HIV-infected adults in the semi-urban district of Entebbe, Eastern Uganda, 25-34 year olds demonstrated the greatest risk for major depressive disorder, with an adjusted OR (OR=4.28) indicating that participants in this age group were more than four times as likely to have MDD than the reference group of 19-24 year olds (Kinyanda, Hoskins, Nakku, Nawaz, & Patel, 2011). Bolton, Wilk, and Ndogoni (2004) yield findings of a more linear nature than the two aforementioned studies, indicating a 1.03 OR increased risk for depression for each additional year of age among adults in rural Uganda. The trend in depression risk related to age is similar among adults from northern Uganda 7 years after the conflict's end. Mugisha et al. (2015) report a steady increase in the odds for depression with each age group, with adults 45 and older demonstrating the greatest risk (OR=2.33 as compared to the reference group of 19-24 year olds).

Considering the association between age and maternal depression in other LMICs, a study conducted by Stewart, Umar, Tomenson, and Creed (2014) in Malawi, a bordering country to Uganda, found no significant association between maternal age and antenatal depression. In a systematic review of the determinants of CMPDs in LMICs, Fisher et al. (2012) conversely found that young age was a significant determinant of these disorders in Nigeria and China in addition to Uganda; however, the remaining majority of the studies included in this review indicated age did not have significant predictive value.

Marital status. The association between marital status and depression postpartum Ugandan women demonstrates no consistent trending across studies in the extant literature. Consistent with much of the greater maternal mental health literature, some studies have found that being married is protective against depression while being single, separated or divorced increases the odds of having postpartum depression (Nakku et al., 2006; Kakyo, Muliira,

Mbalinda, Kizza, & Muliira, 2012). Familiar et al. (2016) identify a similar trend among HIV-infrected female caregivers in Uganda. Kaida and colleagues (2014), however, who analyzed prospective data of HIV-infected women over 7 years through pregnancy, postpartum and non-pregnancy periods, found that never having been married was a protective factor against depression. The analyses published for this study did not identify differential associations of marital status to depression by pregnancy status.Contrary to these findings, however, Kinyanda, Hoskins et al. (2011) found no significant associations between marital status and MDD among HIV-infected individuals.

Importantly, both Kinyanda, Woodburn and others (2011) and Mugisha and colleagues (2015) distinguish participants who had never been married from those who had separated or divorced. In so doing, both research groups found that while separated or divorced participants were about twice (OR=1.95; Mugisha et al., 2015) to three times (OR=3.0; Kinyanda, Woodburn et al., 2011) as likely to have depression than their married or cohabiting counterparts, those who had never been married were about a third (OR=0.3; Kinyanda et al., 2011) to half (OR=0.44; Mugisha et al., 2015) as likely to be depressed, supporting the conclusions made by Kaida and colleagues (2014) that never having married is protective against depression for women. It should be noted, however, that this characteristic of never having been married is specifically identified by puerperal women participating in a qualitative study in Eastern Uganda as a primary contributor to the perceived illness representations of perinatal depression in this community rather than protection against these disorders (Sarkar et al., 2018).

An additional important consideration for the association of marital status with depression is the type of marital structure in which a woman participates, a factor that is often overlooked in these studies. Abbo and colleagues (2008) are perhaps the only authors to investigate marital structure as a correlate of depression among women in Uganda. In this study, married women with co-wives were more than three times as likely (OR=3.65) to demonstrate psychological distress than those who were the only wife to their husband (Abbo et al., 2008). A polygamous marital structure has important implications for the volume of resources, social support, and relationship quality available to a woman. Further research is necessary to assess how this type of arrangement may be contributing to the prevalence of maternal depression among women in Uganda.

Socioeconomic factors. The literature on the socioeconomic risk and protective factors specific to this population are discussed below.

Education. Similar to maternal age, educational attainment is rarely listed among the factors significantly associated with depression in maternal mental health studies (Nakku, Nakasi, & Mirembe, 2006; Kakyo, Muliira, Mbalinda, Kizza, & Muliira, 2012; Familiar et al., 2016). These insignificant findings are consistent with those of studies from other African countries (Abiodun, 2006; Adewuya et al. 2005; Agoub et al. 2005; Adewuya, Eegunranti & Lawal, 2005; Alami et al., 2006; Cooper et al. 1999; Fatoye et al. 2006). One study on urban South African women found that higher levels of maternal education were associated with a lower risk of postpartum depression (Ramchandani et al. 2009). Studies of depression within the general population, however, have yielded mixed findings for education's association with depression. In a study of Ugandan parents of primary school-age children, Huang and colleagues (Huang, Abura, Theise & Nakigudde, 2017) not only found that depression prevalence was higher among female compared to male parents (32% and 9%, respectively), but also among

those with less educational attainment (primary or less education; 41%) compared to those with a

secondary education or greater (18%). Parents who had completed primary school or less were

more than three times as likely (OR=3.15) to have parental depression than their more educated

counterparts (Huang, Abura, Theise & Nakigudde, 2017).

Kinyanda, Woodburn et al. (2011) found evidence to support Huang and colleagues'

finding in a community-based survey covering 14 districts of rural Uganda. Female participants

possessing no formal education within this sample were more than twice as likely (OR=2.2) to

have probable major depressive disorder (PMDD) compared to those who had attained a formal

education. Interestingly, the same lead author in a separate study found no association between

educational attainment and MDD within an HIV-infected sample of adults residing in the semi-

urban district of Entebbe in Uganda (Kinyanda, Hoskins et al., 2011). The overall prevalence of

MDD for this study was 8.1%, a considerably lower percentage than that of Kinyanda,

Woodburn et al.'s (2011) study in rural Uganda, which had a prevalence for PMDD of 29.3%.

Despite their HIV-infection, the sample in Entebbe demonstrated a lower rate of depressive

symptomatology, perhaps due to greater access to resources such as healthcare and education

(Kinyanda, Hoskins et al., 2011). Indeed, the majority of participants in this sample (89.4%) had

acquired at least 7 years of formal education (Kinyanda, Hoskins et al., 2011). Although

Kinyanda, Woodburn and others (2011) did not publish socio-demographic or economic

characteristics for the entire sample, the authors did indicate that only 49.2% of those with

PMDD in the rural Uganda study had attained formal education, a considerably smaller

percentage than that of the semi-urban study. Among district level exposure factors, Kinyanda,

Woodburn and colleagues (2011) found that literacy rate, too, was significantly negatively associated with PMDD, meaning the less literate a participant, the more likely she was to have PMDD.

Familiar and colleagues' (2016) investigation of depression and anxiety among HIV-infected female caregivers of children 2 to 5 years old further obscures the relationship between education and depression. Despite the study's methodological similarities to that of Kinyanda, Woodburn, and others' 2011 study (i.e., similar setting in rural Uganda, use of the same instrument HSCL-25 to screen for depression), Familiar et al. (2016) failed to find a significant association between educational attainment and depression as Kinyanda, Woodburn et al. (2011) had done. A possible explanation for these disparate findings across studies is the role HIV-related factors play in explaining the variance within the relationship of depression and its determinants. As the studies with a sample comprised solely of HIV-infected individuals failed to find significance of education in association with depression, participants with this condition may have depressive symptoms which derive primarily from issues related to their HIV status, while their uninfected counterparts are more readily impacted by their sociodemographic and socioeconomic characteristics.

Socioeconomic status. The extant literature presents a somewhat clearer picture of socioeconomic status (SES) as a risk factor for depression in Uganda. In a study that investigated the effects of a variety of social factors on perinatal depression in rural Uganda, Sarkar and colleagues (2018) found that SES factors such as lack of food and basic needs such as bedding were linked to perinatal depression. By contrast, Nakku, Nakasi & Mirembe (2006) found no significant correlations between SES, measured by house size, and postpartum depression. The authors postulate that the disproportionate inclusion of low SES women utilizing the free public

health facilities at which their participants were recruited may have biased their results.Among

female caregivers (98% of this sample was comprised of biological mothers) of young children,

Familiar et al. (2016) found that being in the top 20% or middle 60% of the wealth index was

protective against depression when compared to individuals falling in the bottom 20% of this

index. Kinyanda, Woodburn et al. (2011) and Abbo et al. (2008) yielded similar findings in the

general Ugandan population. The former group of authors found that one's protection against

PMDD increased with social class (Kinyanda, Woodburn et al., 2011), and the latter identified

participants in debt as being more than twice as likely (OR=2.5) to exhibit psychological distress

(Abbo et al., 2008).

Employment status. The significance of employment status as a correlate for depression

is in dispute and appears to receive little attention in the current literature. Among postpartum

women, female caregivers and within the general population in Uganda, some studies have found

no significant association of employment status with depression (Kakyo, Muliira, Mbalinda,

Kizza, & Muliira, 2012; Kinyanda, Hoskins et al., 2011; Familiar et al., 2016). Kinyanda,

Woodburn and colleagues (2011) and Mugisha et al. (2015) both found, however, that being

employed or being a student made one half as likely or less to be depressed compared to their

unemployed counterparts, indicating that having employment or school enrollment is protective

against depression within the general Ugandan population.

Food security. Across all studies found in the current literature review investigating food

security as a risk factor for depression in Uganda, lack of food increased the odds of an individual presenting with depression (Natamba et al., 2017; Mugisha et al., 2015; Huang et al., 2017; Kinyanda, Hoskins et al., 2011; Abbo et al., 2008). Among both HIV-infected and uninfected adults, food insecurity tends to elevate the risk for depression by two- or three-fold, with odds ratios hovering between 1.99 (Mugisha et al., 2015) and 2.89 (Kinyanda, Hoskins et al., 2011). Risk for depression in the context of food insecurity is, perhaps, the greatest for parents. Huang et al. (2017) found that the parents of families who were food insecure were more than 11 times as likely (OR=11.84) to have parental depression compared to their food secure counterparts.

Adverse life events. The experience of adverse life events is an additional factor with unequivocal significance in association with depression in Uganda. Adverse life events typically include the experience of rape, war-related trauma or torture, the death of a loved one, and severe illness in studies in this country. A number of studies have found the risk for depression to increase predictably as participants endorse a greater number of life events in the previous 12 months (Mugisha et al., 2015; Kinyanda, Hoskins et al., 2011; Kinyanda, Woodburn et al., 2011). The elevated risk for PMDD becomes more pronounced among women when they have endorsed the experience of childhood-related negative life events, particularly the death of their father (Kinyanda, Hoskins et al., 2011). Females in this sample reporting 11 or greater adverse life events in the past year were over 16 times (OR=16.67) as likely to have depression compared to women in this study who reported0 events.

Among pregnant women, Natamba and colleagues (2017) found that those who had experienced domestic violence, resided in a camp for internally displaced persons, or reported experiencing abduction were more likely to have higher depression scores. Among postpartum women, Nakku, Nakasi and Mirembe (2006) found the death of an immediate family member was the adverse life event most frequently experienced in the previous 12 months. The experience of adverse life events was associated with a twofold increase in the odds of postpartum depression in this sample.

Psychosocial factors. The literature on the psychosocial factors associated with depression in this population are explored below.

Intimate partner characteristics. A number of studies in Uganda report dissatisfaction with marriage and lack of support from husband as significant risk factors for postpartum depression. Results from a study conducted in Kabarole District of western Uganda evidenced positive associations between scores on the Edinburgh Postnatal Depression Scale (EPDS) and husband's number of other female sexual partners and current problems in the marriage (Kakyo, Muliira, Mbalinda, Kizza, & Muliira, 2012). A systematic review evaluating the magnitude of postpartum symptomatology offers results corroborating marital conflict as a risk factor for postpartum depression across developed and developing countries (Norhayati et al., 2015).

Ugandan women also directly report unsupportive husbands as a primary contributor to their depression, as indicated through the findings of a rapid ethnographic assessment conducted in eastern Uganda (Tol et al., 2018). In this study, perinatal women participants identified "sickness of thoughts," a local idiom of distress with associated symptoms significantly overlapping with those of perinatal depression, as the most salient mental health issue among pregnant and postpartum women. Perinatal women participants cited absent or unsupportive partners as the most common cause for sickness of thoughts, asserting that the lack of emotional, social or financial support increases the likelihood of a woman in the community developing the condition. Participants additionally reported domestic violence and marital conflicts as causes for sickness of thoughts. The findings from Tol et al. (2018) are corroborated by the conclusions of a qualitative study conducted by Sarkar et al. (2018), who found partner-related issues were cited most often as the primary cause of postpartum depression by perinatal women and local maternal health stakeholders in rural Ugandan settings. Partner-related issues consisted of intimate partner violence, lack of financial provision from the husband, and lack of love from the husband. Using participants from a sub-study conducted in rural Uganda that focused on perinatal depression among women with HIV, Ashaba, Kaida, Coleman, Burns, et al. (2017) found that one major challenge faced during the perinatal period was intimate partner violence, particularly if the pregnancy was unintended.

Family and social relationships. According to the qualitative findings from Tol and colleagues (2018), perinatal Ugandan women most readily find social support outside of their intimate partner relationships from family members and community members such as friends, traditional healers, religious leaders and community health workers. Prayer was emphasized as a primary act of support to assist women dealing with perinatal depression (Tol et al., 2018). Sarkar et al. (2018) found mistreatment and abuse by in-laws, lack of interaction with one's parents, and loneliness to be social factors to increase risk for perinatal depression in rural Ugandan women. Among post-conflict adults in northern Uganda, too, low social support was found to increase the odds of having MDD (Mugisha et al., 2015). Familiar and colleagues (2016) highlight an important interaction, however, reporting that greater family support was more protective against depression when participants were in the highest wealth group index compared to the lowest within a sample of female caregivers to 2- to 5- year-old children in Uganda. This may indicate the role of social support as a complementary buffer against depression, while being materially resourced has the main effect.

Additional psychosocial factors to consider when evaluating risk for depression are the number of children a woman has and the quality of her relationships with them. In a study of psychological distress in Eastern Uganda, Abbo and colleagues (2008) found that persons with more than four children were three times as likely (OR=3.0) to exhibit psychological distress. It should also be noted that single parenthood can increase the odds of depression (OR=1.7; Kinyanda, Woodburn et al., 2011). Finally, Huang and colleagues (2017) found that having a conflicted parent-child relationship and being a proponent of corporal punishment were both associated with a greater depression score among parents in Uganda.

Health factors. The literature on the health factors associated with depression in this population are explored below.

Reproductive health. Perhaps unexpected, factors related to reproductive health tend to lack significance in association with maternal depression. Kakyo et al. (2012) conduct the most rigorous investigation of these factors as they relate to postpartum depression. Among their participants, they failed to find a significant association between depression and any of reproductive health-related factors, including number of past abortions, type of delivery for most recent pregnancy, place of delivery, and the experience of obstetric or postpartum complications (Kakyo, Muliira, Mbalinda, Kizza, & Muliira, 2012). Nakku, Nakasi, & Mirembe (2006)

23

similarly fail to find a significant association between obstetric history or physical problems during pregnancy. The researchers did find, however, that unplanned pregnancy was associated with postpartum depression (Nakku, Nakasi & Mirembe, 2006).

General physical health. As previously discussed, HIV infection makes a significant contribution to the occurrence of maternal depression. Okeke and Wagner (2013) write about the impact of ART on mental health in Ugandan HIV patients, finding that 12 months of ART led to prevalence of inor depression dropping about 15% and prevalence of major depression dropping about 27% compared to a control that did not receive ART. ART also helps close the gender gap in depression. Weiser, Gupta, Tsai, Frongillo, et al. (2012) find that 3 years of ART leads to an improvement in physical health status, among other factors. In a similar vein, Wagner, Ghosh-Dastidar, Garnett, Kityo, & Mugyenyi (2012) discuss the positive impact 12 months of ART have on mental health, noting improvements in depression and reductions in hopelessness and internalized stigma. Despite these disproportionate odds against HIV-infected women, however, Kaida and colleagues (2014) do identify some protective factors against postpartum depression in this population, including increased time on antiretroviral therapy, viral suppression and better physical health.

Within the general population as well, being HIV positive is associated with an increased risk for MDD (Mugisha et al., 2015). Of note, neither Familiar and colleagues (2016) nor Kinyanda, Hoskins and others (2011) found a significant association between antiretroviral treatment status and depression among HIV-infected adults. This may be indicative of the impact of knowing one has HIV and the stigma associated with having this illness on psychological well-being. The shame or alienation of this positive status may overpower the hope of receiving treatment for the condition. Even beyond HIV, Nakku, Nakasi, & Mirembe (2006) found in the study of depression at six weeks postpartum that the endorsement of any current physical illness by a mother was positively associated with postpartum depression.

Reproductive outcomes and infant characteristics. Consideration of the contribution of reproductive outcomes and infant characteristics to maternal depression is understudied in Uganda. In addition to reproductive health, Kakyo and colleagues (2012) have produced the most thorough analyses of these factors. In their computation of obstetric and infant characteristics, the authors found positive correlations between mothers' perceptions of their infants' ability to breastfeed and postpartum depression. They found that parity (the number of viable pregnancies a mother has experienced) was negatively associated with the condition, meaning the fewer pregnancies a woman experienced, the lower her depression score (Kakyo, Muliira, Mbalinda, Kizza, & Muliira, 2012), a finding corroborated by Natamba and colleagues (2017). Factors with associations failing to reach significance in Kakyo and colleagues' (2012) study included maternal and infant complications during childbirth; infant characteristics such as age, sex, weight at birth, current weight or health problems; and giving birth to a baby of the desired sex (Kakyo, Muliira, Mbalinda, Kizza, & Muliira, 2012). In alignment with these findings, Natamba et al. (2017) found no association between postpartum depression and gestational age, and Nakku, Nakasi and Mirembe (2006) reported finding no significant associations between infant sex and low birth weight. The latter research group did find, however, that giving birth to a child of an undesired sex (OR=2.62) and physical problems in the child (OR=2.28) made a woman more than twice as likely to have postpartum depression.

Mental health history. Although neither past treatment for mental illness nor family history of mental illness were associated with major depression among postpartum mothers (Nakku, Nakasi, & Mirembe, 2006), both of these factors were found to be significantly associated with MDD among HIV-infected and post-conflict adults in Uganda (Kinyanda, Hoskins et al., 2011; Mugisha et al., 2015). More specifically, the following psychiatric illnesses were identified as significantly associated with MDD in both populations: alcohol dependency disorder, generalized anxiety disorder, and life-time attempted suicide (Kinyanda, Hoskins et al., 2011; Mugisha et al., 2015). Both studies also identified positive coping style as a protective factor against MDD.

Consequences of Postpartum Depression

As maternal depression is consequential to the health of both mother and child, the repercussions associated with this major global mental health issue are explored below.

Impact of postpartum depression on maternal health. In a qualitative study exploring the contributions of social factors to perinatal depression in Uganda, Sarkar et al. (2018) gather perspectives from community stakeholders on the impact of perinatal depression on a mother. The authors acknowledged that this was a topic of less substantial discussion among participants, a pattern reflected in the greater maternal mental health literature as well, where the health of the mother appears to be a lesser priority than that of the child. In Sarkar and colleagues' (2018) qualitative assessment, interview participants most readily identified the prospect of self-injury or suicide risk as threats to maternal health as a consequence of maternal depression. In a recent systematic review of the impact of maternal depression on maternal and child health outcomes in

LMICS, Surkan, Patel and Rahman (2016) also identified suicidal ideation and self-harm as major consequences of perinatal depression, with ideation prevalence ranging from 4 to 14% across South Asian, South American and SSA countries. The review identified limited healthcare seeking among depressed mothers as a second consequential domain to maternal health (Surkan, Patel, & Rahman, 2016). The authors cite scarcity of mental health services in LMICs and the stigma associated with mental health conditions as barriers to healthcare treatment among perinatal women in these regions (Surkan, Patel, & Rahman, 2016).

Even in high-income countries, the effects of maternal depression on maternal health is understudied. Brown and Lumley (2000), however, are able to shed some light on this relationship in Australia. The researchers found that at 6-7 months postpartum, depression was significantly associated with back pain, sexual problems, digestive issues, relationship issues, tiredness, urinary incontinence, and greater incidence of minor illness. At follow up, the association of poorer emotional wellbeing and the latter three health-related issues persisted (Brown and Lumley, 2000).

Impact of postpartum depression on child health. The study of the effects of maternal depression on child health outcomes, conversely, is steadily rising in both high- and low-income countries. The systematic review conducted by Surkan, Patel and Rahman (2016) identifies effects of maternal stress and depression in utero, on birth outcomes, and in early parenting practices affecting child growth and development as well. The review identifies a number of effects of maternal depression on fetal development, including elevated baseline heart rates, increased heart rate activity, and below average weight of fetuses of depressed mothers (Surkan,

Patel, & Rahman, 2016). Concerning birth outcomes, one study included in this review identified smaller head and abdominal circumferences among the newborns of depressed mothers (Surkan, Patel, & Rahman, 2016).

In a study with children of depressed South African mothers done 18 and 36 months after birth, Garman, Cois, Tomlinson, Rotheram-Borus, and Lund (2019) offer additional evidence for negative consequences of maternal depression on child health. At 18 months, children of mothers who suffer from depression both 6 and 18 months postpartum have significantly lower weight-to-length and weight-for-age z-scores compared to mothers who suffered from prenatal depression but whose EPDS scores decreased after birth - the control group. At 36 months, children of mothers who suffer from depression 18 months after birth had lower weight-for-age z-scores compared to children whose mothers' EPDS scores decreased after birth. Children of mothers who suffered from depression 6 months after birth had significantly lower length-for-age and weight-for-age z-scores compared to the control group.

Maternal depression additionally has adverse effects on mothers' parenting of their infants, which leads to the poor physical and cognitive development of their children, sometimes resulting in death. Hanlon (2013) effectively summarizes associations between maternal depression and these infant outcomes, citing infant undernutrition and diarrhea as particularly consequential to child health. The author identifies delayed breastfeeding initiation as a potential contributor to these adverse effects (Hanlon, 2013). Bennett, Schott, Krutikova, and Behrman (2015) present analyses on data collected from a multicountry longitudinal study of child poverty in four LMICs to support Hanlon's report. The authors found significant associations between maternal mental health in the first year of a child's life and increased risk of poor growth and cognitive development in India and Vietnam (Bennett et al., 2015). The children of depressed mothers in India also demonstrated an elevated risk for poor cognitive development, and children of depressed mothers in Ethiopia demonstrated poor life satisfaction at 8 years of age, indicating persistent and long-term consequences of exposure to poor maternal mental health for child outcomes (Bennett et al., 2015).

Returning to maternal depression in Uganda, Ashaba and colleagues (Ashaba, Rukundo, Beinempaka, Ntaro & LeBlanc, 2015) found a significant association between maternal depression and malnutrition, even after controlling for sociodemographic and economic factors such as education, family size and income source. Among mothers of malnourished children, the prevalence of maternal depression was 42% while among mothers of children with average nutritional status but carrying other chronic conditions had a prevalence of 12% for depression. As the data collected for this study was cross-sectional, directionality of the relationship between maternal depression and these child outcomes could not be determined.

Impact of Maternal Depression on Maternal Practices Promoting Child Health and Nutrition

As previously discussed, the extant literature on the relationship between maternal mental health and maternal child health-promoting practices is severely limited, particularly among LMIC populations, emphasizing the demonstrated need for the current study. Although current research on infant and young child feeding practices are primarily derived from samples in HICs (Daniels et al., 2015; Goulding et al., 2014; Elias et al., 2016; Bronte-Tinkew et al., 2007; Ramsay et al., 2002), some of these insights are transferable to the study of the impact of maternal depression on these behaviors in the SSA context. Hurley, Black, Papas and Caufield (2008) have found that maternal depressive symptomatology is significantly associated with maladaptive feeding of young children. Maternal depressive symptoms have also been linked to reduced breastfeeding initiation, ineffective breastfeeding practices and early termination of breastfeeding (Henderson et al., 2003; Cooper, Murray & Stein, 1993; Grigoriadis et al, 2013).

In an intervention study focused on the improvement of maternal mental health and child development through providing education on parenting practices, Singla, Kumbakumba, and Aboud (2015) found that mothers in the control arm demonstrated an average dietary diversity score of 2.06 out of 7, indicating that children in rural Uganda may not be receiving the balanced, nutritional diet required for normative child growth and development. Sanitation and hygiene practices are a behavioral category more readily studied in SSA countries, but there are currently no studies reporting findings on these practices as they relate to maternal depression. In a multisite study of toilet possession, disposal of child feces in Kenya, Tanzania and Uganda, Tumwine et al. (2003) found that though toilet ownership ranged between 92 and 99.5% across these countries (95% rate in Uganda), over 30% of these toilets were contaminated with feces in rural Uganda, indicating that residents of these areas would benefit from education and support around sanitation and hygiene. In a study conducted by the same author group in these three countries on domestic water use, the authors noted an elevated prevalence of diarrhea (Tumwine et al., 2002). Study results identified determinants of unsafe disposal of feces and wastewater and the use of water obtained from unsanitary sources as the cause of this diarrheal morbidity. Findings from Chung et al. (2004) among low-income women in the United States are also of value to the current study, indicating that mothers with maternal depression were less likely to engage in important infant health practices such as use of the infant back sleep position.

Perceived Social Support, Maternal Depression and Child Health

While it is common for the global mental health literature to present inconsistent findings on the nature of depressive disorders, there is little dispute about the profound mitigating effect social support has upon symptom severity. Across geographic regions and economic strata, the extent of a woman's perceived social support has reliably demonstrated significant associations with the occurrence of maternal depression, where the higher a woman perceived social support from family, friends and significant others, the lower the likelihood of depression (Vaezi, Soojoodi, Tehrani, Banihashemi, & Nojomi, 2018; Pao, Guintivano, Santos, & Meltzer-Brody, 2018; Yagmur & Ulukoca, 2010; Pingo, van den Heuvel, Vythylingum, & Seedat, 2017; Reid & Taylor, 2015).

Contextualized within the relationship between maternal depression and child health and behavior, too, social support appears to play a key role (Lee, Halpern, Hertz-Picciotto, Martin, & Suchindrarn, 2005; McManus & Poehlmann, 2012). McManus and Poehlman yielded findings in a US-based study that the interaction of clinical levels of depressive symptoms at 9 months postpartum and mothers' report of low social support was associated with lower cognitive functioning in their children at 16 months (2011). Their failure to identify depression alone as a significant predictor of a child's cognitive trajectory bolsters the argument for examining mothers' social support as a key determinant of child health. Lee and others (2011) find that

31

social support plays a similar modifying role in maternal depressive symptoms' relation to externalizing behavior issues among children up to 36 months old.

Through structural equation modeling, Herwig, Wirtz and Bengel (2003) seek to partially explain the impacts of depression and social support on child behavior. Both variables indirectly impacted the outcome of child behavior issues through their strong correlations with partnership and parenting, the two factors demonstrating direct impacts on the outcome variable. These findings exemplify not only the critical importance of maternal depression on a child's overall health and wellbeing, but they indicate the utility of social support as a tool for creating an environment for a mother to set her child's life on an upward trajectory and the crucial role an intimate partner plays in the health of both the mother and child.

In Sub-Saharan Africa, especially, a mother's perceived social support is of particular consequence due to its strong associations with important physical health and nutrition indicators for women and their children (Hadley, Mulder, & Fitzherbert, 2007; Field, Onah, van Heyningen, & Honikman, 2018).

This relationship is especially salient in the SSA region, where perceived social support from an intimate partner is commonly shown to carry more weight than support from other sources (Wolf & Frese, 2018). Stewart, Umar, Tomensen and Creed (2014) found that a lower score on the Significant Other subscale of the Multidimensional Scale for Perceived Social Support (MSPSS) exclusively was associated with antenatal depression among Chichewa and Chiyao pregnant women in Malawi; they found no such association between these women's perceived support from family and friends. Importantly, the experience of intimate partner violence (IPV) is a particularly salient variable, as it often informs the relationship between intimate partner violence (IPV) and maternal depression (Field, Onah, van Heyningen, & Honikman, 2018).

Women's Empowerment in the Context of Maternal Depression and Child Health

Despite a growing body of literature investigating the impact of empowering women on their communities, the pool of research evaluating how women's empowerment affects pregnancy, the incidence of maternal depression, and the condition's relationship to critical child health outcomes remains quite small. This literature is particularly underwhelming in the context of LMICs. This section explores emerging trends in the current literature on women's empowerment, which may inform how this construct impacts the interplay between maternal depression and child health outcomes.

Women's Empowerment, Autonomy and Status

While the terms women's empowerment, women's autonomy, and women's status are often erroneously conflated in the literature, each carries important distinctions within its definition and operationalization. While women's autonomy is widely described as a woman's ability to act independently, control her environment and make decisions in her own interests and that of her loved ones (Dyson & Moore, 1983; Jejeebhoy & Sathar, 2001; Basu, 1992; Bloom, Wypij & Gupta, 2001), women's empowerment is believed to cast a wider net, inclusive, too, of the power, status and access to resources that a woman may experience through interdependence, and as a result of greater cultural relevance to those who place higher value on interdependence than independence (Kabeer, 1998; Govindasamy & Malhotra, 1996; Malhotra and Mather, 1997; Mishra & Tripathi, 2011). While women's status clarifies the general position or social standing of women within their society/community (Bloom, Wypij & Gupta, 2001; Mason, 1986; Govindasamy & Malhotra, 1996), the term women's empowerment is designed to capture the advancement or progress women have made in holding power or authority within their households and communities (Kabeer, 2001; Malhotra & Schuler, 2005).

The most readily acknowledged and cited definition of women's empowerment is offered through the seminal work of Naila Kabeer (2001), who conceptualizes empowerment as a person's expanded ability to make life choices where this ability was previously denied them. Kabeer deconstructs empowerment into three dimensions, each of which informs the next; those are resources, agency, and achievements (Kabeer, 1999). She defines resources, which she and others have described as the pre-conditions or "enabling factors" for empowerment, as both material or economic resources, social capital, and political influence (Kabeer, 2001; Malhotra & Schuler, 2005). Mahmud, Shah and Becker (2012) identify education, paid employment, and media exposure as example indicators of a woman's resources.

These authors are careful to emphasize that while the availability of these resources is a prerequisite for the next dimension, a woman's agency, the mere availability of these resources does not equate to having agency, described not only as a woman's access to resources but additionally her ability to control and make use of these resources (Mahmud, Shah & Becker, 2012). Kabeer describes this agency dimension not as a static trait but as a process through which a woman takes advantage of her available resources and experiences empowerment (Kabeer, 1999). Malhotra & Schuler (2005) stress Kabeer's point by emphasizing that what sets women's empowerment apart from other concepts is its encompassing of the process of change and the woman's role as an agent of change within it. As captured in Kabeer's description, empowerment indicates an advancement toward greater freedom of choice and action for persons who did not previously possess such power. Malhotra & Schuler (2005) add, however, that what it means to be empowered is for the woman herself to serve as an actor within that process of change rather than a mere beneficiary.

Finally, resources and agency culminate in what Kabeer describes as achievements, the outcome of empowerment, or a woman's potential to live the life that she wants (Kabeer, 1999). The Oxford Poverty and Human Development Index (Alkire et al., 2013) identify five domains in which a woman can reach "adequate achievement," including decisions about agricultural production, access to and decisions-making power about productive resources, control of use of income, leadership in the community and time allocation.

Women's Empowerment in Sub-Saharan Africa

While the study of women's empowerment has made great strides in the last 3 decades, the construct's applicability has not been uniform across regions. Indeed, the Demographic and Health Surveys (DHS), the largest existing survey program designed to collect nationally representative demographic and health information from LMICs, initiated data collection on WE in 1990 with the addition of a women's questionnaire to its core instrument (Moore & Croft, 1990); its development, however, was informed primarily by WE studies taking place in Asia (Upadhyay & Karasek, 2012). As a result, studies attempting to measure empowerment in sub-saharan African countries have found that some of the most salient indicators of women's empowerment within Asian cultures do not translate easily to women who in SSA countries (Upadhyay and Karasek, 2012; Schatz and Williams, 2012). Heckert and Fabic (2013) gather perspectives from researchers critical of the DHS women's empowerment domain who assert

that empowerment is expressed differently among women in Africa compared to women in Asia,

who are often less mobile, have lesser visibility in public spaces, and exhibit lesser financial

independence (Kishor & Subaiya, 2008). Findings from Upadhyay and Karasek (2012) in their

investigation of the impact of women's empowerment on reproductive outcomes in SSA

countries offer support for these claims. In an effort to understand the insignificance of

household decision-making as an indicator for women's autonomy in three of four SSA countries

studied, the authors posit that decision-making may not play as meaningful a role in the

empowerment and autonomy of women in Africa as it does in Asia. Their findings instead

indicated that attitudes toward gender roles shed more light on the effects of empowerment on a

woman's likelihood of bearing her preferred number of children.

While traditionally meaningful indicators of WE have failed to add explanatory value to

trends within the SSA context, developing a deeper understanding of these domains of WE is of

great consequence, especially as they relate to maternal and infant healthcare services. Sub-

Saharan Africa has been found to be the region suffering the highest rates of maternal and infant

mortality, the unfortunate keeper of about half of these deaths each year (Lawn & Kerber, 2006;

Kinney et al., 2010); this is in part a tragic consequence of underutilization of healthcare

services. Studies evaluating culturally relevant dimensions of empowerment within SSA have

demonstrated the construct is positively associated with maternal, infant and child healthcare and

negatively associated with crucial malnutrition indicators such as stunting (Ewerling et al., 2017;

Pratley, 2016). Heckert and Fabic (2013) bring light to the gaps in information on WE within

SSA.

By interviewing global and country-specific gender and health experts on the WE data and literature of four SSA countries, these researchers identify three primary areas for further study on this construct: economic empowerment, knowledge of legal rights, and participation in decision making. Experts are careful to highlight that differences in cultural or group-level values may cast a long shadow over the attitudes of the individual; as a result, they emphasize the importance of gauging the value-system and support of women at the community level to offer a fuller picture of WE to emerge (Heckert & Fabic, 2013). Additionally, the experts included in this study together issue a charge for data collection on the attitudes and expectations not just of women but also of adolescent girls, the families of women, and their greater communities (Heckert & Fabic, 2013).

Bandiera and others (2015) respond to this charge by means of a randomized controlled trial designed to assess the impact of kickstarting women's empowerment in adolescence through targeted programming for 14-20-year-old females in Uganda. Following 2 years of social and economic empowerment programming offered through voluntary participation in vocational training and education on sex, marriage and reproduction, participants in the intervention arm saw a 72% increase in engagement with income-generating activities, a 25% drop in teen pregnancy and a 58% decrease in early cohabitation compared to baseline rates (Bandiera et al., 2015). Based on the Bangladesh Rural Advancement Committee's (BRAC) gender empowerment programme, the authors emphasize the model's transferability to Uganda and other SSA countries with modifications; they fail to articulate the nature of these modifications, however, and how the results of their program evaluation differ from BRAC's program findings in South Asia. Despite this oversight, Bandiera and colleagues' findings that focused programming on vocational skills, financial literacy, sex and reproductive education, and legal rights in sexual and marital relationships yields considerable increases in the aforementioned WE indicators is consistent with the domains for further study highlighted by Heckert and Fabic's expert interviewees (Bandiera et al, 2015; Heckert & Fabic, 2013).

The developers of the Survey-based Women's Empowerment index (SWPER) also make significant contributions to bridging the gap between lack of meaningful information about WE within the SSA context and available data on this topic. They achieve this through utilization of DHS data to develop an index based exclusively on the data of 34 African countries, 32 of which are SSA (Ewerling et al., 2017). This team employed data-driven processes to arrive at three domains of WE most significant to these cultures: social independence, attitudes toward violence, and decision making. Their findings indicated that attitudes toward violence and decision making were consistently associated with modern contraceptive use while social independence (a domain of the SWPER index capturing educational attainment, ages at first birth and first cohabitation, media exposure, and educational and age differences between a woman and her husband) was linked to institutional delivery and negatively associated with child stunting (Ewerling et al., 2017).

Findings from Adjiwanou and Legrand (2014) similarly convey the importance of attitudes toward violence as a relevant WE domain in SSA, finding that a higher tolerance toward violence against women is associated with a lesser likelihood of skilled birth attendance use across four African countries. Contrary to Ewerling and colleagues, however, they find that decision-making bears no meaningful impact on maternal health care use in these countries.

Women's Empowerment, Maternal Depression and Maternal and Child Health

Issues of women's empowerment become especially salient in the context of the perinatal period, when a woman's physiological and psychosocial vulnerabilities are often heightened. These vulnerabilities can lead to irrevocable consequences for the reproductive, psychological and physical health of both mother and child, including underutilization of care services, maternal mental illness, maternal morbidity and mortality, and the same outcomes for their infants (Will, Khavjou, Finkelstein, Loo, & Gregory-Mercado, 2007; Hindin, 2012; Kyomuhendo, 2003).

In Uganda, specifically, Kyomuhendo (2003) documents the disempowerment that pregnancy can inflict on rural Ugandan women, which results in sorely reduced rates of professional ante- and postnatal healthcare services and institutional delivery. Despite 60% of women surveyed for this study knowing of at least one woman who had died due to obstetric complications in the last year and common knowledge that traditional birthing practices are most used in this area, most reported a distrust of local health facilities, in large part due to poor treatment by health workers (Kyomuhendo, 2003). Participants who had experience with antenatal care or institutional delivery reported feeling they were treated like passive patients, that their preferred cultural practices related to emotional expression and delivery position were undermined, and that their reports of labor and birthing pains went unconsidered (Kyomuhendo, 2003). Health workers interviewed in this same study corroborated these women's views of how they are perceived, reporting beliefs that mothers in this community were ignorant (Kyomuhendo, 2003). The disempowerment these study participants experienced during their pregnancy explained their preference for traditional birthing practices despite their awareness that these birthing attendants are typically unqualified and frequently lead to maternal death

(Kyomuhendo, 2003). Hindin (2012), too, reinforces the risks of disempowerment during this

critical perinatal period in the broader SSA context through a meta-analysis of DHS data in 25

countries. She illustrates the ripple effect that pregnancy-related disempowerment can have on

future WE, finding that pregnancy at an earlier age is associated with poorer expectations of

marital quality and greater belief in wife-beating justifications (Hindin, 2012).

Barber and Gertler (2009) provide insight into how these outcomes could be different

when WE increases. Their findings indicate that an empowerment intervention including cash

transferal directly to women, education about reproductive health and services, and self-

advocacy training leads to increased prenatal healthcare consumption compared to non-

participants in this intervention (Barber & Gertler, 2009). Indeed, in the broader context of

women's health, empowerment is additionally associated with reduced rates of unintended

pregnancy (Upadhyay et al., 2014), reduced rates of sexually-transmitted infection within high-

risk populations (Shain et al., 1999), and lower glucose and cholesterol levels among women

presenting with high risk for diabetes and cardiovascular disease (Will, Khavjou, Finkelstein,

Loo, & Gregory-Mercado, 2007).

With the awareness that perinatal depression can further complicate the health outcomes

of women and their children, empowering women can serve as a protective and potential

mitigating factor against perinatal depression and its many negative consequences, which, as

aforementioned, include maternal self-injury and suicide risk (Sarkar et al., 2018), elevated

baseline heart rate and activity and low birth weight among fetuses and infants (Surkan, Patel, &

Rahman, 2016), below-average head circumference among infants (Surkan, Patel, & Rahman,

2016), delayed breastfeeding initiation (Hanlon, 2008), increased risk of poor growth and cognitive development, and poorer life satisfaction among children of depressed mothers (Bennett et al., 2015).

Although it remains small, the body of literature on the relationship between mental health and women's empowerment has experienced recent growth as experts in the global mental health and maternal and child health fields begin to recognize its importance. Further research is required to better understand how one construct informs the other. While findings from Baranov, Bhalotra, Biroli and Maselko (2017) indicate that perinatal depression is a crucial component of women's empowerment, and intervention at this level is critical for disrupting the continuity of gender inequality across generations, the authors acknowledge that clarifying the directionality of the association between maternal depression and issues of women's disempowerment is a difficult task. Baranov and colleagues' acknowledgement is further supported by the qualitative report of Kermode et al.'s (2007) study, which summarizes the conceptualizations of mental health and illness among women in rural India. These conceptualizations are inextricably fused with prominent dimensions of women's empowerment, including autonomous decision-making; high status within the household, the extended family and the community; freedom of movement; and the freedom from intimate partner violence (Kermode et al., 2007).

The successful findings of interventions for depression assessing WE outcomes and others intervening at the WE level to assess effects on maternal depression may indicate that identifying the direction of this relationship may be unimportant. The Thinking Healthy Program intervention implemented as a highly effective treatment for antenatal depression additionally yielded long-lasting effects on WE domains for its participants 7 years after implementation

(Baranov, Bhalotra, Biroli & Maselko, 2017). The impacts of this treatment for depression on women's empowerment included increased financial empowerment, increased control over household financial decisions, and increased time and financial investment in children, particularly when the child was female (Baranov, Bhalotra, Biroli & Maselko, 2017).

Garcia and Yim (2017) gather evidence from 10 studies evaluating a variety of maternal and parental empowerment interventions reporting on perinatal depressive symptoms. The authors found that seven of the 10 studies resulted in a reduction of perinatal depressive symptoms. The same systematic review reported the findings of 11 empowerment intervention studies evaluating pre-term birth and low birthweight as outcomes. All 11 studies yielded positive effects of the intervention on these outcomes, with two of these studies reporting additional benefits for gestational age (Garcia and Yim, 2017).

That the authors of this systematic review were unable to identify any studies reporting on the impact of women's empowerment on both perinatal depression and the aforementioned child health outcomes highlights a gap in the extant literature. There is little understanding of how women's empowerment informs the crucial relationship between maternal depression and child health. With the previously established awareness that eliminating maternal depression would reduce the prevalence of child underweight and stunting—conditions belaboring SSA more than any other region in the world—by close to 30%, it is imperative that the mitigation of the impact of perinatal depression is at task approached from every possible angle.

The Current Study

The purpose of the current study is to explore in a sample of Ugandan mothers of children less than 24 months old how maternal behaviors affecting child health differ in the presence or absence of maternal depression and to explore how perceived social support and women's empowerment and autonomy may moderate the relationship between maternal depression and mothers' engagement in these behaviors. This study addresses the gaps in the literature through quantifying the specific impact maternal depression can have on the uptake of maternal behaviors known to affect child health. While there is currently a wealth of evidence from LMICs supporting the existence of a relationship between maternal depression and child health outcomes, there is little exploration of the underlying mechanisms through which maternal depression operates to impact children's nutritional status. Through careful investigation of the uptake of specific behavioral indicators (behavior categories include care seeking for sick children; infant and young child feeding practices; water, sanitation and hygiene; and child illness prevention practices) known to affect child health outcomes in both depressed and nondepressed mothers, the current study offers a valuable contribution to the extant literature on the effects of maternal depression. This knowledge would prove useful in directing researchers, policy makers and relief and development programmers toward the behaviors most significantly impacted by maternal depression as they work to optimize their programming for maximum impact.

Additionally, the current study explores the potential moderating effects of perceived social support and women's empowerment and autonomy to the relationship between maternal depression and the uptake of these important, health-promoting behaviors. Understanding the effects of these constructs could offer additional approaches for targeting maternal depression, a primary global health issue (Surkan et al., 2011).

Aims and Hypotheses

The study's purpose of exploring the impact of probable depression on mothers' self-report of behaviors promoting child health will be explored through the following aims and hypotheses:

Aim 1. To examine the psychometric properties of the Patient Health Questionnaire-9 (PHQ-9) and Multidimensional Scale of Perceived Social Support (MSPSS) as they pertain specifically to the current sample.

Aim 1a. To examine the psychometric properties of the Luo version of the PHQ-9 in the current sample of northern Ugandan women.

Hypothesis 1a. The PHQ-9 will retain its original unidimensional factor structure in the current sample of northern Ugandan women.

Aim 1b. To examine the psychometric properties of the Luo version of the MSPSS in the current sample of northern Ugandan women.

Hypothesis 1b. The factor structure of the MSPSS will retain its original three-factor structure (Factor groups: (1) social support from family; (2) social support from friends; (3) social support from significant other) in the current sample of northern Ugandan women.

Aim 2. To critically assess differences between probably depressed and nondepressed mothers in their endorsement of child health promoting behaviors and in child health outcomes.

Aim 2a. To critically assess how mothers' endorsement of behaviors promoting child health differ in probably depressed and nondepressed mothers with at least one child less than 24 months of age. The behavior domains to be evaluated include the following:

(1) Integrated management of childhood illness

(2) Infant and young child feeding practices

(3) Water, sanitation and hygiene behaviors

(4) Child illness prevention practices.

Hypothesis 2a. Seeking advice or treatment for child illness within 24 hours and knowledge of at least three signs of childhood illness that require immediate treatment will be **negatively** associated with maternal depression.

Hypothesis 2b. Provision of more breast milk or fluid to ill children, the same amount or more food than usual to 6-23-month-old ill children, exclusive breastfeeding of children younger than 6 months and minimum dietary diversity for children 6-23 months will be **negatively** associated with probable depression.

Hypothesis 2c. Availability of a soap and water hand-washing station in the home, safe disposal of child fecal matter, and use of an adequate treatment method of household drinking water will be **negatively** associated with probable depression.

Hypothesis 2d. Mothers' use of an insecticide-treated mosquito net for children 0 -23 months will be **negatively** associated with probable depression.

Aim 2b. To critically assess differences in child health outcomes (child underweight, defined as weight-for-age Z score greater than two SDs below the mean, and child stunting, defined as height-for-age Z score greater than two SDs below the mean) between the index children of probably depressed and nondepressed mothers.

Hypothesis 2e. Child underweight will be **positively** associated with probable depression.

Hypothesis 2f. Child stunting will be **positively** associated with probable depression.

Aim 3. To investigate the impact of mothers' perceived social support on (1) the relationship between maternal depression and mothers' demonstration of behaviors affecting child health; (2) the relationship between maternal depression and the prevalence of child underweight (as measured by weight-by-age Z-score); and (3) the relationship between maternal depression and the prevalence of child stunting (as measured by height-by-age Z-score).

Hypothesis 3a. Mothers' perceived social support will moderate the relationship between maternal depression and uptake of maternal behaviors affecting child health.

Hypothesis 3b. Mothers' perceived social support will moderate the relationship between maternal depression and the prevalence of child underweight.

Hypothesis 3c. Mothers' perceived social support will moderate the relationship between maternal depression and the prevalence of child stunting.

Aim 4. To investigate the impact of mothers' perceived empowerment (as measured by indicators of household decision-making, attitudes toward intimate partner violence, and contraception use) on (1) the relationship between maternal depression and maternal uptake of behaviors affecting child health; (2) the relationship between maternal depression and the prevalence of child underweight (as measured by weight-by-age Z-score), and (3) the relationship between maternal depression and the prevalence of child stunting (as measured by height-by-age Z-score).

Hypothesis 4a. Mothers' perceived empowerment will moderate the relationship between maternal depression and uptake of maternal behaviors affecting child health.

Hypothesis 4b. Mothers' perceived empowerment will moderate the relationship between maternal depression and the prevalence of child underweight.

Hypothesis 4c. Mothers' perceived empowerment will moderate the relationship between maternal depression and the prevalence of child stunting.

CHAPTER III

METHOD

Setting

The current study utilized pre-existing, cross-sectional baseline data from the aforementioned parent project. The baseline data for this project were collected in Kitgum District of Northern Uganda, an area severely devastated by the armed conflict brought on by the Lord's Resistance Army and other rebel movements from 1986 to 2005, which resulted in the internal displacement and economic plundering of millions of Ugandans living in Kitgum and other northern districts and consequently, enduring poverty in the region compared to the rest of the country (Green, Blattman, Jamison & Annan, 2016; Uganda Ministry of Finance, Planning and Development, 2003). Kitgum district therefore demonstrates staggering rates for depression (24.7%; Mugisha, Muyinda, Malamba & Kinyanda, 2015). The study's catchment area includes 6 (Labongo Amida, Lagoro, Labongo Akwang, Kitgum Matidi, Labongo Layamo, Omiya Anyima) of the 10 sub-counties in Kitgum District. According to the National Population and Housing Census of 2014, Kitgum District has a population of about 204,000, about 104,800 of whom are female (Uganda Bureau of Statistics, 2017). The 6 sub-counties included in the study catchment area were then divided into clusters, each containing about 120 households. Forty-three of these clusters were randomly selected for inclusion in the study.

Participants and Procedure

For all 43 randomly selected clusters, one pregnant woman and/or mother of at least one child under 24 months of age from each household was approached by independent enumerators, affiliated with neither Teachers College nor our study partners Food for the Hungry or Johns Hopkins University, for participation in the parent study.

Having a child under 24 months was an inclusion criterion for this study due to substantial evidence supporting the importance of the first 1000 days of a child's development (conception to 24 months) in predicting the cognitive and physical health trajectories of that child across his lifespan (Schwarzenberg & Georgieff, 2018; Rogers, Manges, Finlay & Prendergrast, 2019; Cusick & Goergieff, 2016; Kattula et al., 2014; De Onis & Branca, 2016). Exclusion criteria included exhibiting current and elevated risk for suicide and/or another acute mental health condition (e.g., bipolar disorder, psychosis), and being under 18 years of age.

Due to previously reported illiteracy rates of close to 50% among women in Kitgum district, enumerators obtained informed consent by reading the consent form to each person to be screened. If a respondent verbally consented to participation in the baseline interview, she either signed or thumb-printed the consent form. The following demographic information was collected from all consenting respondents: respondent name and age; language(s) spoken; preferred language; whether the respondent was pregnant at the time of interviewing, and the name, date of birth, and sex of their child under 24 months. Respondents were then screened for depressive symptoms using the Patient Health Questionnaire-9 (PHQ-9), an instrument commonly used to screen for depression and validated for use in Uganda (Kroenke, Spitzer & Willians, 2001; Akena, Joska, Obuku, & Stein, 2013; Nakku et al., 2016).

49

Item 9 on the PHQ-9 assesses frequency of thoughts of suicide or self-harm ("In the last week, how often have you been bothered by thoughts that you would be better off dead, or of hurting yourself?") in the patient; a respondent may select("Not at all"), 1 ("1 to 3 days"), 2 ("4 to 5 days"), or 3 ("6 to 7 days"). To measure clinical severity of a response larger than zero , the research team for the parent study developed a protocol to ensure appropriate follow-up, and if necessary, referral, to a higher level of clinical care for cases involving suicidality. The suicide prevention protocol included administration of the Columbia Suicide Severity Rating Scale (C-SSRS) if a respondent selected a response greater than zero on item 9 of the PHQ-9 (Posner et al., 2008). The C-SSRS assesses severity of suicidality on three levels: low risk, moderate risk, and high risk (Posner et al., 2008). With the permission of the primary author of the tool, changes were made to the measure in response to feedback on the measure's acceptability from promoters during the pre-trial training. The language was simplified, and the date of the most recent suicide attempt was recorded to track risk for a future attempt. Respondents who demonstrated moderate to high risk of suicide based on results of the C-SSRS were referred to one of the five regional mental health clinics of the Health Rights International organization (formerly the Peter C. Alderman Foundation).

An overview of the sampling procedure is presented in Figure 1. In total, 3489 respondents completed these components of the baseline interview. If a respondent consented to participation, met eligibility criteria and met criteria for probable depression, assessed by use of a modified algorithm, her interview continued, and she completed the full baseline interview. One thousand three hundred forty two of these 3489 respondents (referred to as Round 1 respondents) met these requirements and were thus recruited into the parent study. If a respondent met exclusion criteria or their PHQ-9 responses did not indicate probable depression according to the aforementioned algorithm, they were thanked and did not continue with the complete baseline survey (called "non-complete respondents"). Two thousand one hundred forty-seven respondents fell into this category. These Round 1 interviews were conducted from September 7, 2017 to November 8, 2017.

After the first round of baseline interviewing concluded in November 2017, it was decided that a small portion of the respondents who did not meet criteria for probable depression should be approached to complete the full baseline interview for the purpose of comparing depressed and nondepressed women. This second round of baseline interviewing was carried out from November 14 to December 22, 2017. A convenience sample of 328 of the 2147 non-complete respondents were therefore approached a second time to complete the full baseline survey during a second round of interviewing, carried out. The 328 women who completed a baseline interview during this second round are referred to as "Round 2 respondents." The current study utilized the data from the completed interviews of Round 1 ($n = 1028$) and Round 2 respondents ($n = 284$), for a total sample of 1312 respondents.

A total of 358 additional respondents were excluded from the current analyses due to exclusion criteria. This included 298 respondents who were excluded from the current analyses due to having no children under 24 months of age at the time of interviewing, which reduced the sample of Round 1 respondents to 1079 and Round 2 respondents to 293. Forty-four additional respondents were excluded (Round 1: $n = 1040$; Round 2: $n = 288$) from analyses due to male gender. Four adoptive mothers and three grandmothers found in Round 1 only were excluded because they were not the biological mother to the index child (Round 1: $n = 1033$). Nine additional cases were excluded from Rounds 1 and 2 due to incomplete or inconsistent data. This

resulted in an updated sample size of 1312 (Round 1: $n = 1028$; Round 2: $n = 284$).

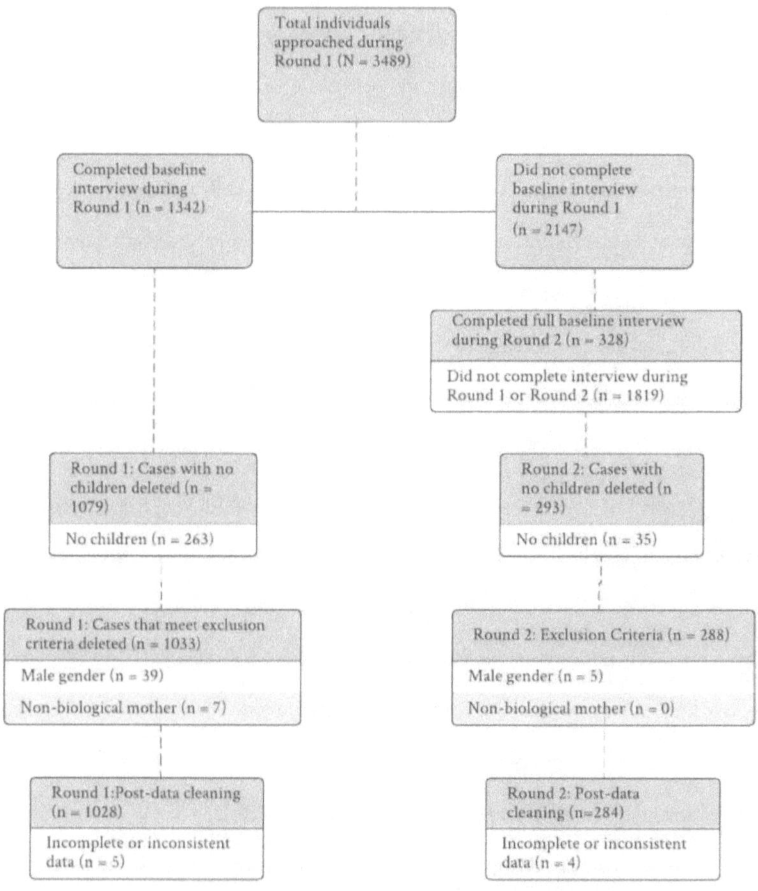

Figure 1: Overview of Sampling Procedure

Measures

Sociodemographic Variables

Sociodemographic variables of the respondents were collected within the baseline survey questionnaire. The information collected included sub-county and parish of residence, languages spoken, maternal age, characteristics of an index child between 0 and 23 months of age (child age, sex, and date of birth), pregnancy status, maternal gender, marital status and religion.

Household composition. Household characteristics were also collected during the baseline interview, including the following: number of family members in household, number of biological children under 5 years, number of children under 5 years living in the household, whether biological children and biological father are living in the home, and head of household.

Socioeconomic variables. Socioeconomic variables collected included educational attainment (i.e., number of years of school attended), literacy (assessed through the respondent reading part or the whole of two sentences written in the local language for the enumerator), employment status, type of employment, hours per day respondent spends away from index child, and other caregivers of index child. A household dietary diversity index was also administered, which collects information on the consumption of foods from a variety of different food groups by any household member in the previous 24-hour period. The Household Dietary Diversity (HDD) score serves as a proxy for household socioeconomic status, a practice supported by the multicountry findings of Hoddinot and Yohannes (2002).

Probable depression status. Symptoms of maternal depression were assessed using the Patient Health Questionnaire-9 (PHQ-9), a depression screening tool previously validated for use

53

in Uganda (Akena, Joska, Obuku, & Stein, 2013; Nakku et al., 2016) and among postpartum women in other SSA settings (Weobong et al., 2008; Green et al., 2018). It was recommended by mental health professionals from the region to reduce the time period of 2 weeks covered by this measure to1 week due to their determination that it is unlikely for women in this region to effectively recall frequency of symptoms in the last 2 weeks in the manner that the PHQ-9 requires. The questionnaire was therefore modified such that respondents were asked to answer items according to the previous week rather than 2 weeks. Because this modification falls short of the 2-week time specifier delineated by the DSM-V for a depressive disorder, this measure is defined as probable depression (American Psychiatric Association, 2013).

Additionally, local mental health professionals anticipated the language used for the response options of the PHQ-9 (i.e., "Not at all," "Several days," "More than half the days," and "Nearly every day") would not be found acceptable in this community. These response options were therefore made more concrete, presenting these response options in days. The response option "Not at all" was therefore changed to "0 days," "several days" to "1 to 3 days," "more than half the days" to " 4 to 5 days," and "nearly every day" to "6 to 7 days" (See Appendix A).

Suicide risk. Respondent risk for suicide was assessed using the Columbia Suicide Severity Rating Scale (C-SSRS), which was administered if a respondent endorsed a response greater than zero on item 9 of the PHQ-9, which screens for suicidal ideation. With the permission of the primary author of the C-SSRS (Posner et al., 2008), minor changes in wording were made to simplify the language of the measure, an action taken in response to feedback from local IPT-G promoters who participated in the IPT-G training.

Integrated management of childhood illness. The baseline survey included items from the

Water, Sanitation and Hygiene (WASH) module of the Knowledge, Practices and Coverage

(KPC) survey (Monitoring, C.O.R.E., & Evaluation Working Group, 1999). The KPC is a widely

used and highly adaptable tool used for the planning, monitoring and evaluation of maternal and

child survival programs (Child Survival Support Project, Macro International, CORE Group,

MCHIP, & MCSP, 2016). The KPC includes eight technical modules from which researchers

can draw to create household surveys tailored to the community of study. Information on

integrated management of childhood illness (IMCI) was collected using items from the Sick

Child module of the KPC survey. The questions included in the baseline questionnaire from this

module pertained to the indicators of care-seeking for a sick child and maternal knowledge of

danger signs of childhood illness. A mother waws considered to demonstrate adequate

knowledge when she could spontaneously list three or more danger signs. This cutoff is informed

by the recommendations for this indicator by USAID's Measure Evaluation (MEASURE

Evaluation Project, 2017).

    Water, sanitation and hygiene behaviors. The questions included in the baseline

questionnaire from the WASH module pertained to the following indicators: household water

treatment, soap-and-water handwashing station in the household, and safe disposal of feces.

    Infant and young child feeding practices. Information on respondents' infant and

young child feeding practices (IYCF) were collected using items from the Nutrition module of

the KPC survey. The questions included in the baseline questionnaire from this module pertained

to the following indicators: exclusive breastfeeding under 6 months, continued breastfeeding at1year, minimum acceptable diet, frequency of complementary feeding, and provision of fortified and nutrient-dense complementary foods.

Child illness prevention practices. Information on mothers' child illness prevention practices was collected using items from the Immunization and Malaria modules of the KPC survey. The questions included in the baseline questionnaire from this module pertained to the indicators of growth monitoring, immunization, Vitamin A supplement issuance, and long-lasting insecticide net ownership and use by children.

Women's empowerment and autonomy. Women's empowerment and autonomy has been assessed through inclusion of the following indicators from the Gender and Family Planning and Birth Spacing modules of the KPC as well as the Women's Empowerment module of the Demographic and Health (DHS) surveys, and some of which are also represented in the Survey-based Women's Empowerment Index (SWPER): attitudes toward intimate partner violence, respondent's participation in household decision-making, and use of contraception. Attitudes toward IPV was identified by Asaolu et al. (2018), in their exploratory and confirmatory factor analyses of women's empowerment indicators as the most persistent factor of women's empowerment across all regions of SSA, which included East Africa. Based on DHS data from 34 SSA countries, the SWPER identified attitudes toward IPV and household decision-making as two of its the three domains (Ewerling et al., 2017). Relevant data were unavailable from the current sample to include the SWPER's final domain, social independence.

Perceived social support. Perceived social support was assessed using the Multidimensional Scale of Perceived Social Support (MSPSS; Zimet, Dahlem, Zimet & Farley, 1988). This instrument features three subscales, measuring perceived social support from a respondent's (1) significant other, (2) family, and (3) friends. It has previously been translated into Luganda and validated for use in a southern Ugandan setting among postpartum mothers (Nakigudde, Musisi, Ehnvall, Airaksinen & Agren, 2009). Informed by both Nakigudde and colleagues' (2009) adaptation of the MSPSS tool and the input of our northern Ugandan care group and mental health providers, the 7-point likert scale the original MSPSS instrument utilizes was collapsed into a 2-tiered, dichotomized response option model (i.e., Participants were first given the "agree" or "disagree" response options, followed by "agree a little/agree a lot" or "disagree a little/disagree a lot" based on the initial response). Both sources indicated that due to the high illiteracy rates in the study population, it was likely that the 7-point likert scale would demonstrate poor acceptability and be difficult to understand. This alternative model was adopted to reduce the number of distinctions participants would need to make between response options.

Child health status. Child nutritional status was assessed through the anthropometric measurement of children 6-23 months of age (height, weight), following the protocol outlined in the Nutrition module of the KPC. Weight-for-age and height-for-age Z-score variables were generated using the WHO Anthro Survey Analyser macro for SPSS, which calculates these scores based on WHO child growth standards (WHO, 2009). Outcomes for child health status were underweight (low weight-for-age) and stunting (low height-for-age), which were defined by Z-scores greater than two standard deviations below the mean for weight-for-age and height-for-age, respectively.

Human Subjects Approval

Data for the current study were collected by Food for the Hungry with the ethical approval of the Teachers College, Columbia University Institutional Review Board. National approval to collect these data in Uganda was granted by the Uganda National Council for Science and Technology, and regional approval was granted by the Gulu University Research Ethics Committee. As the current study analyzes archival data collected from the baseline time point of the parent project and programmatic data collected for Food for the Hungry Care Group programming, it produces minimal risk exposure for its participants.

Data Analysis

Using SPSS, descriptive statistics were first calculated to assess for significant differences in sociodemographic and economic characteristics between depressed and nondepressed participants. The variables included in this analysis were the following: subcounty and parish of residence, maternal age, characteristics of an index child between 0 and 23 months of age (child age, sex, and date of birth), number of biological children, pregnancy status, marital status, religion, household composition characteristics, educational attainment, literacy, employment status, and household dietary diversity score.

Aim 1. To evaluate the psychometric properties of the Multidimensional Scale of Perceived Social Support and Patient Health Questionnaire-9, reliability analyses, exploratory factor analyses, and confirmatory factor analyses were conducted for each instrument. The random-split half sample procedure was used for factor analyses, informed by the recommendation of Anderson and Gerbing (1988). These analyses were performed using JASP version 0.13.1.

 Aim 2. To assess how rates of demonstrated behaviors affecting child health differ in depressed and nondepressed mothers with at least one child under 24 months of age across behavior categories (integrated management of child illness, infant and young child feeding practices, water, sanitation and hygiene behaviors, and child illness prevention behaviors), bivariate analyses (chi-square and non-parametric Mann Whitney U-tests) were first run using SPSS version 26.0 to assess for differential rates of demonstrated behaviors between depressed and nondepressed participants. Based on the results of these analyses, a series of logistic regressions and penalized regressions were run using SPSS version 26.0 to provide odds-ratios on the likelihood of a mother demonstrating each behavioral indicator, based on probable depression status (probably depressed or not depressed). Hierarchical multiple regressions were run for continuous outcome variables to determine the effects of probable depression status above and beyond relevant covariates.

 Aim 3. To investigate the impact of mothers' perceived social support on (1) the relationship between maternal depression and maternal uptake of behaviors affecting child health; (2) the relationship between maternal depression and the prevalence of child underweight (as measured by weight-by-age Z-score), and (3) the relationship between maternal depression and the prevalence of child stunting (as measured by height-by-age Z-score), a series of multiple logistic and multiple linear regressions were performed, including mean MSPSS score as a moderator in these analyses. These analyses were run using SPSS.

Aim 4. To investigate the impact of mothers' perceived autonomy on (1) the relationship between maternal depression and maternal uptake of behaviors affecting child health; (2) the relationship between maternal depression and the prevalence of child underweight (as measured by weight-by-age Z-score), and (3) the relationship between maternal depression and the prevalence of child stunting (as measured by height-by-age Z-score), a series of logistic and hierarchical linear regressions were run, where the composite scores of household decision-making, attitudes toward intimate partner violence and contraception use were each included as moderators of these analyses. These analyses were run using SPSS.

CHAPTER IV

RESULTS

Preliminary Analyses

Data Preparation

Because the study sample includes data from two rounds of interviewing completed about 2 months apart, preliminary analyses were performed to summarize the data collected during the first and second rounds of interviewing, and comparison analyses were performed to determine whether the data from Round 2 is representative of the pool of respondents who did not complete interviews in Round 1.

Comparing non-complete respondents and Round 2 respondents. Because only a portion of participants who did not complete interviews due to lower PHQ-9 scores in Round 1 were selected for interviewing in Round 2, it was important to determine whether the respondents selected for Round 2 interviewing were representative of the larger sample of non-complete respondents from which they were drawn. To achieve this, tests of independence were run to determine if there were significant differences between non-completers and Round 2 respondents in all demographic variables that non-complete respondents completed, as well as total PHQ-9 scores.

For categorical variables, chi-square tests of independence were run. For continuous variables, normality was assessed for both non-complete and Round 2 samples through visual inspection of each variable's histogram and corresponding P-P plots and tests of significance for skewness and kurtosis (Skewness and kurtosis scores were converted to z-scores. Values exceeding 1.96 were considered to deviate significantly from the expected values of a normal

61

distribution at $p < 0.05$; Field, 2013). Because data for all continuous variables included in these analyses did not follow a normal distribution but were similar in shape for both samples, nonparametric Mann-Whitney U-tests were performed to determine whether there were statistically significant differences between non-complete and Round 2 samples.

Demographic variables. A statistically significant difference was found for the sub-county in which the respondent resides ($\chi^2(5) = 16.20$, $p = .007$, Cramer's V = .087). The associations of this variable to interview round was small (Cohen, 1988). These significant results were expected due to the convenience sampling method employed to interview Round 2 respondents. No statistically significant differences were found between the two groups for any of the remaining demographic variables, including respondent age ($U = 298642.50$, $z = .03$, $p = .941$), age of the index child ($U = 1807380.0$, $z = -0.21$, $p = .830$), or number of children under 24 months, $\chi^2(3) = 2.94$, $p = .401$, Cramer's V = .037 (See Table 1).

PHQ-9 score. No statistically significant differences were found between non-complete respondents and Round 2 respondents in PHQ-9 score ($U = 280642.0$, $z = -0.89$, $p = .376$; See Table 1). Because no statistically significant differences were found neither for total PHQ-9 score nor most demographic variables, and strength of associations were small for those with significant differences, use of the Round 2 respondents as a representative sample of all respondents who did not complete the full interview during Round 1 was considered appropriate.

Table 1

Summary of Participant Demographics and PHQ-9 Score for Non-Complete and Round 2 Respondents

| | Interview Round | | | | | | |
| Measure | Non-complete (n = 1819) | | Round 2 (n = 328) | | Total Sample (n =2147) | | Test Statistic |
	n	*%*	*n*	*%*	*N*	*%*	
Subcounty							$\chi^2 = 16.20**$
Kitgum Matidi	427	23.5	64	19.5	491	22.9	
Labongo Akwang	250	13.7	64	19.5	314	14.6	
Labongo Amida	189	10.4	19	5.8	208	9.7	
Labongo Layamo	256	14.1	42	12.8	298	13.9	
Lagoro	214	11.8	39	11.9	253	11.8	
Omiya Anyima	483	26.6	100	30.5	583	27.2	
Languages Spoken							$\chi^2 = 2.56$
Luo	1816	99.8	328	100	2144	99.9	
English	288	15.8	51	15.5	339	15.8	
Other	67	3.7	7	2.1	74	3.4	
Pregnancy Status (Pregnant)	429	23.6	67	20.4	496	23.1	$\chi^2 = 1.56$
Number of children < 24 mos.							$\chi^2 = 2.94†$
0 children	417	22.9	68	20.7	485	22.6	
1 child	1381	75.9	259	79.0	1640	76.4	
2 children	13	1.0	1	0.3	19	0.9	
3 children	3	0.2	0	0	3	0.1	
Index child sex							$\chi^2 = 0.86$
Male	719	39.5	136	41.5	855	39.9	
Female	683	37.5	124	37.8	807	37.6	
No children	417	22.9	68	20.7	481	22.4	
	Mean *(SD)*		**Mean *(SD)***		**Mean *(SD)***		
Age	25.72 *(6.14)*		25.73 *(6.19)*		25.72 *(6.15)*		$z = 0.03$
PHQ-9 Score	7.05 *(4.20)*		6.90 *(4.51)*		7.02 *(4.25)*		$z = -0.88$
Index child age (months)	8.40 *(5.20)*		8.33 *(5.20)*		8.39 *(5.20)*		$z = -0.21$

Notes. * $p < .05$ (two-tailed). ** $p < .01$ (two-tailed). *** $p < .001$ (two-tailed).

Descriptive Statistics

Descriptive statistics were calculated for all variables included in analysis. For categorical variables, depressed and nondepressed respondents were compared using chi-square tests of independence. For continuous variables, normality was assessed through visual inspection of each variable's histogram and corresponding P-P plots and tests of significance for skewness and kurtosis (Skewness and kurtosis scores were converted to z-scores. Values exceeding 1.96 were considered to deviate significantly from the expected values of a normal distribution at $p < 0.05$; Field, 2013). Because these assessments indicated that the data for none of the continuous variables were normally distributed, depressed and nondepressed respondents were compared using non-parametric Mann-Whitney U tests. Demographic variables are discussed below. Correlations for all independent variables and continuous outcome variables are presented in Table 2. Descriptive statistics for all test variables are presented as they apply to hypothesis testing in each aim's section.

Demographic variables. A summary of demographics and PHQ-9 scores for depressed and nondepressed participants is presented in Table 3. A Mann-Whitney U test was performed to determine whether there were differences in respondent age between depressed and nondepressed respondents. Distributions of respondent age were similar, as assessed by visual inspection of each group's histogram. Median age was statistically significantly higher in depressed (*Mdn* = 26.00) compared to nondepressed (*Mdn* = 24.00) respondents, $U = 134167.50$, $z = -2.09$, $p = .036$. A statistically significant association was also found between depression and whether a respondent works for income outside the home, ($\chi^2(1) = 122.89$, $p < 0.001$, Cramer's V = .306) which carried a moderately strong association (Cohen, 1988). Of depressed respondents,

41.1% reported performing income-generating work compared to 6.0% of nondepressed

respondents. A statistically significant difference between depressed and nondepressed

participants was also found for the type of work ($\chi^2(5) = 14.67$, $p = .012$, Cramer's V $= .183$)

respondents reported performing. Harvesting work (27.0%) was most frequently reported among

depressed respondents while shop-keeping and/or street vending (29.4%) was most common for

nondepressed respondents. It is important to note that the difference found between depressed

and nondepressed participants who work and their type of work may be attributable to Round 1

and Round 2 interviews taking place in different seasons, which may have caused common work

opportunities like harvesting to no longer be available to respondents at the time of Round 2

interviewing.

No significant difference was found between depressed and nondepressed participants for

literacy level ($\chi^2(2) = .90$, $p = .639$, Cramer's V $= .030$), assessed in accordance with the

Demographic Health Surveys' protocol of marking a respondent "literate" if she is able to read at

least one complete sentence written in the local language and "partially literate" if she reads part

of at least one sentence (Croft et al., 2018). Of depressed participants, 35.5% of those who

attempted ($N = 814$) demonstrated literacy compared to 33.0% of nondepressed respondents who

attempted the literacy test ($N = 203$). Similarly, statistically significant differences between

depressed and nondepressed women were not found for years of education attained. Distributions

of years of education were similar, as assessed by visual inspection of each round's histogram.

Six years was the median for both rounds, $U = 1498249.0$, $z = 1.37$, $p = .172$.

Depressed and nondepressed respondents did not significantly differ in terms of

household dietary diversity (HDD) score, $U = 136508.0$, $z = -1.70$, $p = .089$, the total count of the number of different food groups consumed by a household within the previous 24-hour period. This variable was used as a proxy for socioeconomic status in the current and parent studies. With a possible range of zero to 12, the mean HDD score among depressed respondents was 4.19 (SD = 1.79) and 4.001(SD = 1.78) for nondepressed respondents. Depressed and nondepressed respondents similarly did not significantly differ in religion, $\chi^2(2)$ = 0.54, p = .765, Cramer's V=.020, with Catholicism being most frequently reported for both depressed (68.9%) and nondepressed (68.0%) respondents.

Regarding marital status ($\chi^2(3)$ = 16.79, p < .001; Cramer's V= .113), statistically significant differences were found between rounds, with nearly two-thirds (61.1%) of nondepressed respondents reporting cohabitation with a partner to whom they were not married compared to 51.0% of depressed respondents with this status. Statistically significant differences were also found between depressed and nondepressed respondents for head of household ($\chi^2(4)$ = 21.77, p < .001, Cramer's V = .129). Among depressed respondents, 77.0% reported their husband/partner was head of household while 89.1% of nondepressed respondents reported this household head. Depressed and nondepressed respondents did not statistically significantly differ by pregnancy status ($\chi^2(1)$ = 1.15, p = .284, Cramer's V = .030). Of depressed respondents, 2.9% were pregnant at the time of interviewing compared to 1.8% of nondepressed respondents.

Regarding characteristics of respondents' children (see Table 4), significant differences were found between depressed and nondepressed women for the number of children under 5 years of age living in the respondent's household, U = 125590.5, z = -3.94, p < .001, and how many of those children were the respondent's biological child, U = 130121.0, z = -3.09, p = .002. A median of 2 was found for both depressed and nondepressed participants for both variables.

Depressed and nondepressed women also demonstrated a statistically significant difference in child age, $U = 172284.0$, $z = 4.66$, $p < .001$. Distributions of index child age were similar, as assessed by visual inspection of each group's histogram. Median child age in months was statistically significantly higher for nondepressed mothers (*Mdn* = 11) compared to depressed mothers (*Mdn* = 9). No statistically significantly differences were found between groups for sex of the index child, $\chi^2(1) = .66$, $p = .655$, Cramer's V = .012. The index children of depressed mothers were comprised of 51.8% females compared to 50.3% of their nondepressed counterparts.

A statistically significant difference was found between the depressed and nondepressed groups for the sub-county in which the respondent lives, $\chi^2(5) = 81.29$, $p < .001$, Cramer's V = .249. While residents of Labongo Amida comprised the greatest portion of the depressed sample (23.3%), the highest percentage of nondepressed respondents were from the Omiya Anyima sub-county (33.1%).

Table 2

Correlation Matrix for All Independent and Continuous Variables Included in Analyses

Variable	1	2	3	4	5	6	7	8
1. Depression Status	-							
2. Perceived social support	-.41***$^\perp$	-						
3. Household decision-making	-.20***$^\perp$	.11***	-					
4. Attitudes toward IPV	.27***$^\perp$	-.01	-.20***	-				
5. Contraception use	-	.02$^\perp$	-.05$^\perp$	.05$^\perp$	-			
6. Knowledge of danger signs of child illness	.61***$^\perp$	-.24***	-.15***	.22***	.11***	-		
7. Number of essential nutrition actions	-.20***$^\perp$	.13***	.08*	-.06	.05	-.16***	-	
8. Number of complementary feedings	.11**$^\perp$	.06	.10**	-.07	-.06	-.04	22***	-

Note. All correlation coefficients are Spearman's Rho except $^\perp$ are point biserial.

* *p* < .05 (two-tailed). ** *p* < .01 (two-tailed). *** *p* < .001 (two-tailed).

Demographics and PHQ-9 score for Probably Depressed and Nondepressed Participants

	Depression status						
	Probably Depressed *(n = 1028)*		*Not Depressed* *(n = 284)*		*Total Sample* *(n =1312)*		
Measure	*n*	*%*	*n*	*%*	*N*	*%*	Test Statistic
Employment status (Employed)	422	41.1	17	6.0	439	33.5	χ^2=122.89***
Literacy Level							χ^2= 0.90
Literate	289	35.5	67	33.0	356	35.0	
Partially literate	225	27.6	54	26.6	279	27.4	
Illiterate	300	36.9	82	40.4	382	37.6	
Marital Status (Living w/ partner)	524	51.0	173	61.1	697	53.1	χ^2= 16.79**
Religion (Catholic)	708	68.9	193	68.0	901	68.7	χ^2= 0.54
Household Head							χ^2= 21.54***
Respondent	113	11.0	10	3.5	123	9.4	
Husband/Partner	792	77.0	253	89.1	1045	79.6	
Other	123	12.0	21	7.4	144	11.0	
Subcounty							χ^2= 81.29***
Kitgum Matidi	171	16.6	59	20.8	230	17.5	
Labongo Akwang	160	15.6	52	18.3	212	16.2	
Labongo Amida	240	23.3	16	5.6	256	19.5	
Labongo Layamo	166	16.1	36	12.7	202	15.4	
Lagoro	136	13.2	27	9.5	163	12.4	
Omiya Anyima	155	15.1	94	33.1	249	19.0	
Languages Spoken							χ^2= 2.92
Luo	1027	99.9	284	100	1311	99.9	
English	162	15.8	48	16.9	210	16.0	
Other	37	3.6	5	1.8	42	3.2	
Pregnant	30	2.9	5	1.8	35	2.7	χ^2= 1.15
	Mean *(SD)*		**Mean *(SD)***		**Mean *(SD)***		
Age	27.09 *(6.46)*		26.27 *(6.57)*		26.91 *(6.49)*		z =-2.09*
PHQ-9 Score	17.48 *(3.33)*		2.33 *(2.46)*		14.22 *(6.99)*		z =25.82**
Years of education	5.22 *(2.98)*		5.55 *(2.73)*		5.29 *(2.93)*		z = 1.37
Household Dietary Diversity (HDD)	4.19 *(1.79)*		4.01 *(1.78)*		4.15 *(1.79)*		z = -1.70

Notes. Literacy level determined by ability to read part (partially literate) or all (literate) of at least one test sentence in preferred language.

* $p < .05$ (two-tailed). ** $p < .01$ (two-tailed). *** $p < .001$ (two-tailed).

Table 4

Child Characteristics for Probably Depressed and Nondepressed Participants

Measure	Probably Depressed (n = 1028)		Not Depressed (n = 284)		Total Sample (n =1312)		Test Statistic
	n	*%*	*n*	*%*	*N*	*%*	
Number of children < 24 mos.							χ^2 = 1.19₁
1 child	1012	98.4	282	99.3	1294	98.6	
2 children	16	14.1	2	0.7	18	1.4	
Index child age group							χ^2 = 9.76**
<6 months	333	32.5	73	25.7	406	30.9	
6 – 23 months	694	67.8	212	74.6	906	69.1	
Index child sex							χ^2 = 0.20
Male	495	48.2	141	49.6	636	48.5	
Female	533	51.8	143	50.4	676	51.5	
	Mean *(SD)*		**Mean *(SD)***		**Mean *(SD)***		
Children < 5 in household	2 *(Mdn)*		2 *(Mdn)*		2 *(Mdn)*		z = -3.93***
Biological children < 5	2 *(Mdn)*		2 *(Mdn)*		2 *(Mdn)*		z = -3.09**
Index child age (months)	8.48 *(5.12)*		10.23 *(5.79)*		8.86 *(5.31)*		z = 4.66***

Notes. * $p < .05$ (two-tailed). ** $p < .01$ (two-tailed). *** $p < .001$ (two-tailed).

Aim 1: Psychometric Properties of the Patient Health Questionnaire-9 (PHQ-9) and the

Multidimensional Scale of Perceived Social Support (MSPSS)

While the PHQ-9 and MSPSS have been validated for use in Uganda, these studies were

conducted in Southern Uganda, typically in urban areas surrounding the capital. These scales

have not been assessed for the validity of their use in Northern Uganda, a much more rural

region. In addition, the formatting of both measures was modified to accommodate the current

sample. For the PHQ-9, response options were modified from the original language used to

reflect the number of days a respondent experienced a symptom (e.g., the original response

option of "several days" was changed to "1 to 3. days"). Additionally, participants were asked to

summarize the frequency of their symptoms in the previous week only (See Appendix A). This

contrasts with the formatting of the original version of the PHQ-9, for which each item pertains

to frequency of symptoms in the last 2 weeks. For the MSPSS, the response option structure was

reduced from a 7-point Likert scale to 4-points (See Appendix B). The second aim of this study

evaluates the psychometric properties of both modified measures on this Northern Ugandan

sample.

Psychometric Properties of the PHQ-9

Internal consistency. The reliability of the PHQ-9 scale was assessed using Cronbach's alpha.

The full scale demonstrated a high level of internal consistency, as demonstrated by a

Cronbach's alpha of 0.907.Cronbach-α-if-item-deleted analysis indicated that removal of an item

would result in marginally reductions in internal consistency with the exception of item 9 ("In

the last week, how often have you been bothered by having thoughts that you would be better off dead or of hurting yourself in some way?"), which if dropped would increase the Cronbach's

alpha value of the scale by .004 (Table 5). The mean score for this scale was 15.52 *(SD* = 7.83).

Table 5

Psychometric Properties of the Patient Health Questionnaire-9

Item	M *(SD)*	Cronbach's α if item deleted
Over the last week, how often have you been bothered by the following problems?		
1. Little interest or pleasure in doing things	1.50 *(1.09)*	0.902
2. Feeling down, depressed, or hopeless	1.97 *(1.07)*	0.887
3. Trouble falling or staying asleep, or sleeping too much	1.77 *(1.06)*	0.892
4. Feeling tired or having little energy	1.79 *(1.03)*	0.893
5. Poor appetite or overeating	1.75 *(1.08)*	0.896
6. Feeling bad about yourself—or that you are a failure or have let yourself or your family down	1.70 *(1.12)*	0.894
7. Trouble concentrating on things, such as reading the newspaper or watching television	1.25 *(1.07)*	0.900
8. Moving or speaking so slowly that other people could have noticed. Or the opposite—being so fidgety or restless that you have been moving around a lot more than usual	1.33 *(1.06)*	0.898
9. Thoughts that you would be better off dead, or of hurting yourself	0.78 *(1.03)*	0.910
10. If you checked off any problems, how difficult have these problems made it for you to do your work, take care of things at home, or get along with other people?	1.67 *(0.99)*	0.889

Structural validity. Because the modified version of the PHQ-9 utilized in this study applies to a shorter time period than the original version (See Appendix A), and this measure was used in a different cultural context than it was originally developed, the validity of this measure needed to be assessed for the current sample. Validity of this measure followed the same two-step modeling approach (Anderson and Gerbing, 1988) applied for the MSPSS. Exploratory factor analysis (EFA) was first performed on a random selection of half of the current sample to determine whether a factor structure differing from that of the original PHQ-9 would emerge. A CFA was then run on the second randomly selected sample to confirm the final factor structure identified by the EFA.

Exploratory factor analysis. An exploratory factor analysis (EFA) was run to analyze the underlying factors for the current sample in the PHQ-9 using JASP. Data were screened for multivariate assumptions (normality, linearity, homogeneity, and homoscedasticity), and all assumptions were met. Zero outliers were detected using z-scores. There were a total of two missing values for this scale, the cases for which were excluded pairwise. The following EFA analyses were conducted using guidelines outlined in Preacher and MacCallum (2003).

The current analysis utilized maximum likelihood estimation with direct oblimin rotation due to expected factor correlation. Parallel analysis and visual inspection of a scree plot were in agreement, suggesting one overall factor, which is consistent with the measure's original factor structure. The one-factor structure had good fit, indicated by both the RMSEA at .06, 90% CI [.046, .069] and the TLI of .97 meeting the recommended cutoffs. Factor 1 retained all 10 items of the PHQ-9, and all item loadings were above the recommended .400 cutoff (see table 7).

73

Confirmatory factor analysis. The one-factor EFA model was confirmed using

confirmatory factor analysis. The CFA was run on the second randomly selected subsample of

the data and also utilized maximum likelihood estimation with direct oblimin rotation due to

expected factor correlation. The results of this analysis indicated good fit of the one-factor

model, $\chi^2 35) = 137.40$, $p < .001$. Both the TLI (.96) and CFI (.97) met the recommended cut-off

of .95 or greater, and the RMSEA value (.068) fell below the recommended value of .08 (Hu &

Bentler, 1999; Yuan & Bentler, 1998). Standardized factor loadings for the CFA of the MSPSS

are presented in Table 8. The results of the EFA and CFA for the PHQ-9 demonstrate that the

unidimensional structure of the original version of this measure holds in this northern Ugandan

sample.

Table 6

Goodness-of-Fit Indices for the EFA and CFA of the PHQ-9

	χ^2 (df)	RMSEA (90% CI)	TLI	BIC
EFA (1 factor)	112.52*** (35)	.058 (.046, .069)	.97	-115.44
CFA (1 factor)	137.40*** (35)	.068 (.056, .080)	.96	15867.09

Notes. * $p < .05$ (two-tailed). ** $p < .01$ (two-tailed).
*** $p < .001$ (two-tailed). RMSEA = Root Mean Squared Error of Approximation.
TLI = Tucker Lewis Index. BIC = Bayesian Information Criteria.

Table 7

Loadings for the EFA One-Factor Model of the PHQ-9

Item	Factor 1
1	0.596
2	0.863
3	0.777
4	0.766
5	0.725
6	0.747
7	0.624
8	0.650
9	0.442
10	0.819

Note. Applied rotation method is oblimin.

Table 8

Standardized PHQ-9 Factor Loadings for Confirmatory Factor Analysis

					95% CI	
Item	Std. Loading	Estimate	Std. Error	p-val	Lower	Upper
1	0.658	0.734	0.040	< .001	0.655	0.813
2	0.862	0.922	0.034	< .001	0.854	0.989
3	0.788	0.837	0.036	< .001	0.767	0.907
4	0.726	0.760	0.037	< .001	0.688	0.831
5	0.713	0.762	0.038	< .001	0.688	0.835
6	0.753	0.842	0.039	< .001	0.766	0.917
7	0.560	0.610	0.041	< .001	0.530	0.690
8	0.679	0.731	0.039	< .001	0.656	0.807
9	0.456	0.469	0.040	< .001	0.391	0.548
10	0.843	0.852	0.033	< .001	0.787	0.916

Note. Applied rotation method is oblimin.

Psychometric Properties of the MSPSS

Internal consistency. The reliability of the MSPSS scale and its three subscales (Family, Friends, Significant Others) was assessed using Cronbach's alpha. The full scale demonstrated a high level of internal consistency, as demonstrated by a Cronbach's alpha of 0.89. This level of reliability is maintained for both the probably depressed and nondepressed samples (Table 9). All MSPSS subscales demonstrated acceptable internal consistencies, as shown in Table 9, for nondepressed mothers, depressed mothers and the entire sample. Cronbach-α-if-item-deleted analysis indicated that removal of an item would result in marginal reductions or increases in internal consistency (See Table 10). While the correlations between the Family and Friends and

Family and Significant Other subscales were weakly correlated, the Friends and Significant

Others subscale correlation was of moderate strength (see Table 11). All correlations reached

statistical significance at $p < .005$.

Table 9

Scale Reliability Statistics for the MSPSS

Scale	Total Sample (n = 1312)		Depressed (n = 1028)		Nondepressed (n = 284)	
	M (SD)	Cronbach's α	M (SD)	Cronbach's α	M (SD)	Cronbach's α
Total MSPSS scale	36.84 (8.38)	0.891	35.20 (8.18)	0.873	42.67 (6.23)	0.884
Family subscale	12.40 (3.35)	0.830	11.82 (3.36)	0.813	14.39 (2.41)	0.800
Friends subscale	12.04 (3.25)	0.816	11.50 (3.16)	0.796	14.01 (2.51)	0.796
Significant other subscale	12.48 (3.25)	0.770	11.94 (3.30)	0.752	14.33 (2.24)	0.710

Psychometric Properties of the MSPSS for the Entire Sample

Item	M (SD)	Cronbach's α if item deleted
Family Subscale		
3. My family really tries to help me.	3.01 (1.07)	0.880
4. I get the emotional support I need from my family	3.01 (1.06)	0.879
8. I can talk about my problems with my family	3.25 (0.93)	0.878
11. My family is willing to help me make decisions	3.07 (1.04)	0.877
Friends subscale		
6. My friends really try to help me.	3.03 (0.98)	0.876
7. I can count on my friends when things go wrong.	2.81 (1.11)	0.877
9. I have friends with whom I can share my joys and sorrows.	3.13 (0.95)	0.888
12. I can talk about my problems with my friends.	3.12 (0.91)	0.878
Significant Other Subscale		
1. There is a special person who is around when I am in need.	3.05 (1.07)	0.876
2. There is a special person with whom. I can share my joys and sorrows.	3.18 (1.02)	0.877
5. I have a special person who is a real source of comfort to me.	3.12 (1.06)	0.878
10. There is a special person in my life who cares about my feelings.	3.13 (1.06)	0.877

Table 11

Bivariate Correlations for MSPSS Subscales for Entire Sample (N = 1312)

Subscale	Family Subscale	Friends Subscale	Significant Other Subscale
Family subscale	1		
Friends subscale	.213***	1	
Significant other subscale	.243***	.578***	1

Notes. Spearman correlation.

* $p < .05$ (two-tailed). ** $p < .01$ (two-tailed). *** $p < .001$ (two-tailed).

Structural validity. Because the 7-point likert-scale response options of the original version of the MSPSS were collapsed into 4 points within 2 tiers (See Appendix B), and this measure was used in a different cultural context than it was originally developed, the validity of this measure needed to be assessed. The current study adopted a two-step modeling approach based on the seminal work of Anderson and Gerbing (1988). Exploratory factor analysis (EFA) was first performed on a random selection of half of the current sample to determine whether a factor structure differing from that of the original MSPSS version would emerge given differences in culture and likert-scale response options for this sample. Run on the second randomly selected sample, a confirmatory factor analysis (CFA) followed the EFA to confirm the final factor structure.

Exploratory factor analysis. An exploratory factor analysis (EFA) was used to analyze the underlying factors for the current sample in the MSPSS Scale using JASP. Data were screened for multivariate assumptions (normality, linearity, homogeneity, and homoscedasticity), and all assumptions were met. Zero outliers were detected using *z*-scores. A Missing Completely at Random (MCAR) test was run in SPSS to determine the appropriateness of using multiple imputation. As this test was found to be significant, indicating possible systematic missingness, the multiple imputation method was not utilized and cases with missing values were excluded pairwise. The following EFA analyses were conducted using guidelines outlined in Preacher and MacCallum (2003).

The current analysis utilized maximum likelihood estimation with direct oblimin rotation due to expected factor correlation. Visual inspection of a scree plot suggested three overall factors, which is consistent with the theory upon which the measure's original factor structure is based. Other methods of extraction yielded differing results, however. While parallel analysis indicates two factors, the Kaiser criterion (eigenvalues greater than 1) suggests there is only one factor for the MSPSS scale within this sample. Because the Kaiser criterion is an extraction method for which recent literature considers outdated and offers little support (Matsunaga, 2010; Patil, Singh, Mishra & Donavan, 2008), its suggested factor structure is not represented here. Model fit is evaluated below for the two- and three-factor structures.

Two-factor structure. The two-factor structure achieved simple structure by loading each item on only one factor, though the two-factor structure drops items 1 and 2 using the criterion that loadings must be greater than .400. Reducing this criterion to .300 factor loading returns items 1 and 2 to factor 1 in the two-factor model; however, at this criterion level, item 1 cross-loads onto both factors. The two-factor model had mediocre fit: both the RMSEA at .081, 90%CI [.071, .091] and the TLI of .91 indicates acceptable fit (Table 12). Factor one retained all four items of the Family susbcale from the original version of the MSPSS (items 3, 4, 8 and 11) and also loaded items 5 and 10 (Friends) of the significant other subscale (See Table 13). Both factors demonstrated a high level of reliability, with Chronbach's alpha scores of .829 (Factor 1) and .815 (Factor 2).

  Three-factor structure. The three-factor structure also achieved simple structure, and all 12 items loaded onto the same factors (Family, Friends, Significant Other) as in the original version of the measure. The loadings for the two- and three-factor models are presented in Tables 13 and 14, respectively. The three-factor model demonstrated an improved fit compared to the two-factor structure. The RMSEA indicated moderate fit at .07, 90%CI [.058, .082], while the TLI (.93) more closely approaches the cutoff for good fit than the two-factor model (Table 12).

Table 12

Goodness-of-Fit Indices for EFA of the MSPSS

Model	$\chi^2 (df)$	RMSEA (90% CI)	TLI	BIC
2-factor	231.752*** (43)	0.081 (.071, .091)	.908	-48.317
3-factor	139.330*** (33)	.070 (.058, .081)	.933	-75.606

Notes. * $p < .05$ (two-tailed). ** $p < .01$ (two-tailed).
*** $p < .001$ (two-tailed).
RMSEA = Root Mean Squared Error of Approximation.
TLI = Tucker Lewis Index.
BIC = Bayesian Information Criteria.

Table 13

Loadings for the EFA Two-Factor Model of the MSPSS

Item	Factor 1 (Family and SO)	Factor 2 (Friends)
1	0.349	0.302
2	0.398	0.291
3	**0.761**	-0.059
4	**0.834**	-0.099
5	**0.488**	0.263
6	0.054	**0.711**
7	-0.084	**0.606**
8	**0.561**	0.148
9	0.112	**0.662**
10	**0.463**	0.259
11	**0.639**	0.074
12	-0.039	**0.812**

Note. Applied rotation method is direct oblimin.
Factor loadings are bolded for ease of reading.

Table 14

Loadings for the EFA Three-Factor Model of the MSPSS

Item	Factor 1 (Family)	Factor 2 (Friends)	Factor 3 (Sig. Other)
1	-0.044	0.054	**0.644**
2	-0.013	0.030	**0.677**
3	**0.734**	-0.036	0.037
4	**0.751**	-0.096	0.108
5	0.076	0.000	**0.683**
6	-0.009	**0.633**	0.157
7	-0.041	**0.602**	-0.022
8	**0.608**	0.198	-0.060
9	0.126	**0.654**	0.021
10	0.207	0.106	**0.418**
11	**0.670**	0.118	-0.038
12	-0.010	**0.807**	0.004

Note. Applied rotation method is direct oblimin.
Factor loadings are bolded for ease of reading.

Confirmatory factor analysis. The three-factor EFA model was confirmed using confirmatory factor analysis due to goodness-of-fit indices suggesting three factors better fit these data than two. The CFA was run on the second randomly selected subsample of the data and also utilized maximum likelihood estimation with direct oblimin rotation due to expected factor correlation. The results of this analysis indicated good fit of the three-factor model, $\chi^2(51)$ = 172.48, $p < .001$ (See Table 15). Both the TLI (.95) and CFI (.96) met the cut-off value of .95 or greater, and the RMSEA value (.07) fell below the recommended value of .08 (Hu & Bentler, 1999; Yuan & Bentler, 1998). Standardized factor loadings for the CFA of the MSPSS are presented in Table 16. The results of the EFA and CFA for the MSPSS suggest that the three-factor structure of the original version of this scale is appropriate for this northern Ugandan sample of mothers.

Table 15

Goodness-of-Fit Indices for the CFA of the MSPSS

Model	$\chi^2(df)$	RMSEA (90% CI)	TLI	BIC
3-factor	172.48*** (51)	.066 (.055, .076)	.948	16658.788

Notes. * $p < .05$ (two-tailed). ** $p < .01$ (two-tailed).
*** $p < .001$ (two-tailed).
RMSEA = Root Mean Squared Error of Approximation.
TLI = Tucker Lewis Index.
BIC = Bayesian Information Criteria.

Table 16

Standardized MSPSS Factor Loadings for Confirmatory Factor Analysis

Factor/Item	Std. Loading	Estimate Std. Error		p-val.	95% CI	
					Lower	Upper
Family						
3	0.778	0.828	0.040	< 001	0.749	0.906
4	0.842	0.893	0.038	<.001	0.818	0.968
8	0.697	0.654	0.037	<.001	0.582	0.726
11	0.736	0.794	0.041	<.001	0.713	0.875
Friends						
6	0.777	0.801	0.039	<.001	0.724	0.877
7	0.700	0.777	0.044	<.001	0.691	0.863
9	0.801	0.790	0.037	< 001	0.717	0.863
12	0.745	0.681	0.035	<.001	0.611	0.750
Significant Other						
1	0.599	0.653	0.045	<.001	0.564	0.742
2	0.690	0.696	0.040	<.001	0.617	0.775
5	0.687	0.730	0.043	<.001	0.647	0.814
10	0.713	0.766	0.043	<.001	0.682	0.850

Aim 2: Comparing Rates of Maternal Behaviors Promoting Child Health in Probably Depressed and Nondepressed Mothers

To critically assess how reported rates of maternal behaviors promoting child health differed in probably depressed and nondepressed mothers, a series of chi-square tests of association and non-parametric Mann-Whitney U-tests were carried out. These tests were followed by a series of multivariate multiple and logistic regressions to further define the relationships among these variables. The behavior categories evaluated included the following: (1) Integrated Management of Childhood Illness; (2) Infant and young child feeding practices; (3) Water, sanitation and hygiene behaviors; and (4) Child illness prevention practices. The same analysis procedure was carried out to assess how child underweight and stunting differed in probably depressed and nondepressed mothers.

Integrated Management of Childhood Illness

To examine the bivariate relationships between probable depression status and behaviors in the domain of integrated management of childhood illness, chi-square tests of independence and Mann-Whitney U-tests were run. Probably depressed and nondepressed respondents were found to statistically significantly differ in whether their child had presumable pneumonia/acute respiratory infection in the last 2 weeks, $\chi^2(1) = 17.92$, $p < .001$, when they sought treatment for their child's illness, $\chi^2(1) = 9.96$, $p = .002$, where treatment was sought, $\chi^2(2) = 6.39$, $p = .041$, and their knowledge of three or more danger signs of child illness, $\chi^2(1) = 227.44$, $p < .001$. Treating knowledge of danger signs as a continuous variable also yielded a statistically significant difference. No statistically significant difference was found between groups for whether or not they sought advice or treatment for their child's illness (See Table 17).

A series of logistic and hierarchical multiple regressions were then carried out for the variables with statistically significant results in the tests of differences to determine differential odds for a given behavior between depressed and nondepressed respondents. Covariates for these analyses included participant age, child age, child sex, number of children under 5 years living in the household, marital status, whether the participant is employed, head of household (respondent or other), respondent's years of education, and household dietary diversity score.

A binomial logistic regression was performed to ascertain the effects of probable depression on the likelihood that participants had a child with presumable pneumonia/acute respiratory infection (symptoms of fast or difficult breathing or fever) in the last 2 weeks. The logistic regression model was statistically significant, $\chi^2(10) = 38.80\ p < .001$. The model explained 4.0% (Nagelkerke R^2) of the variance in child illness and correctly classified 57.5% of cases. Probable depression status was a statistically significant predictor of presumable pneumonia/ARI above and beyond the effects of the aforementioned covariates (as shown in Table 18). Probably depressed participants were 79.9% more likely to have had a child with presumable pneumonia in the last 2 weeks (OR = 1.80, 95% C.I.: 1.343, 2.407).

A multinomial logistic regression was carried out to determine whether there were differences between probably depressed and nondepressed mothers in the odds of when they sought treatment for their sick child (within 24 hours, 2 days later, or 3 or more days later). Although the final model was only marginally significant, $\chi^2(20) = 31.25$, $p = .052$, *Nagelkerke* $R^2 = .060$, probable depression status was found to be a significant predictor over and above the effects of the covariates included in the model ($\chi^2(2) = 10.67$, $p = .005$; see Table 19). Compared to probably depressed participants, nondepressed participants were more than three times as

87

likely to seek treatment for their child's illness within 24 hours rather than 3 days or later

(OR=3.788, 95% C.I.: 1.453, 9.901). Probable depression was not a significant predictor when

comparing women who sought treatment for their children 2 days later versus 3 days or more.

The multinomial logistic regression model including where participants sought treatment for

their sick child was also significant, $\chi^2(40) = 100.14$, $p < .001$, *Nagelkerke R^2* = .216; however,

probable depression status did not significantly contribute to the prediction of this outcome

variable, $\chi^2(4) = 6.55$, $p = .162$ (See Table 20).

A binomial logistic regression was run to determine the effects of depression on the

likelihood that participants knew at least three danger signs of childhood illness. The logistic

regression model was statistically significant, $\chi^2(10) = 285.35$ $p < .001$. The model explained

26.5% (Nagelkerke R^2) of the variance in child illness and correctly classified 65.3% of cases.

Probable depression status was a statistically significant predictor of knowledge of three or more

danger signs above and beyond the effects of the aforementioned covariates (see Table 18).

Depressed participants were more than 24 times more likely to know at least three danger signs

compared to their nondepressed counterparts (OR = 24.35, 95% C.I.: 14.25, 41.52).

Due to the small number of nondepressed participants who knew at least three danger

signs of childhood illness and to better understand the role of probable depression in knowing

danger signs, a Poisson regression was run with robust standard errors for parameter estimates to

account for potential violation of the assumption that the variance and mean of the outcome

variable are equal. This test was chosen based on the recommendations for analysis of low count

data and the current data's violation of the multiple regression analysis' assumption of

independence of residuals. See Table 8 for full details on the poisson regression model. The likelihood ratio chi-square test was statistically significant, $\chi^2(10) = 730.28$, $p < .001$. Probable

depression status was significantly associated with the number of danger signs of child illness a

mother knew, $b = 1.54$, $SE = 0.07$, $p < .001$. The incidence rate ratio (found in the Exp(B)

column of Table 21) indicates that the incidence rate of knowledge of danger signs for depressed

mothers was more than four times greater than for nondepressed mothers.

Table 17

*Summary for Tests of Differences in Integrated Management of Childhood Illness (IMCI)
Between Probably Depressed and Non-Depressed Respondents*

	Depression status				
	Probably depressed (n = 1012)		*Not Depressed (n = 282)*		
Measure	*n*	*%*	*n*	*%*	Test Statistic
Index child ARI illness in last 2 weeks	585	57.8	123	43.6	$\chi^2 = 17.92$***
Advice/treatment sought for child illness	535	90.2	113	91.1	$\chi^2 = 0.10$
When treatment was sought					$\chi^2 = 9.96$**
Same or next day	361	67.9	92	82.9	
2 days or later	171	32.1	19	17.1	
Where treatment was sought					
Community distributor	75	20.8	12	13.0	$\chi^2 = 17.95$***
Health center	150	41.6	36	39.1	
Hospital	52	14.4	18	19.6	
Private Clinic	49	13.6	5	5.4	
Other	35	9.7	21	22.8	
Knowledge of 3 or more danger signs of child illness	579	56.3	17	6.0	$\chi^2 = 227.44$***
	Mean *(SD)*		**Mean *(SD)***		
Knowledge of danger signs of child illness	3.35 *(2.32)*		0.74 *(0.92)*		$z = 22.08$***

Notes.
* $p < .05$ (two-tailed). ** $p < .01$ (two-tailed). *** $p < .001$ (two-tailed).

Table 18

Results of Binomial Logistic Regressions for IMCI Behaviors

Variables	Child Illness in the last 2 weeks	Knowledge of 3 or more danger signs
	OR (95% CI)	OR (95% CI)
Probable depression status	1.799 (1.34—2.41)**	24.33 (14.25—41.52)***
Head of Household (respondent)	0.88 (0.58—1.34)	1.02 (0.66—1.58)
Marital status (partnered)	1.01 (0.71—1.55)	1.16 (0.77—1.74)
Employed	1.17 (0.91—1.51)	0.75 (0.58—0.96)*
Index Child Sex (female)	0.88 (0.70—1.10)	1.09 (0.85—1.39)
Respondent age (years	0.99 (0.97—1.01)	1.03 (1.00—1.05)*
Index Child Age	1.05 (1.02—1.07)**	1.02 (0.99—1.04)
Number of children < 5 years	1.11 (0.95—1.30)	0.96 (0.82—1.13)
Education	1.00 (0.96—1.04)	1.01 (0.97—1.06)
Household Dietary Diversity Score	0.98 (0.91—1.05)	1.06 (0.99—1.14)

*Note. *p < .05. **p < .01. ***p < .001.*

Results of the Multinomial Logistic Regression for When Treatment Was Sought for Child Illness

Variable	Same or next day vs. Three or more days later (reference)		Two days later vs. Three or more days later (reference)	
	Odds	95% CI	Odds	95% CI
Probable depression status	**.264**	**.101—.688**	.405	.134—1.220
Head of Household (respondent)	.736	.305—1.775	.479	.145—1.580
Marital status (partnered)	.429	.155—1.185	.534	.163—1.753
Employed	1.127	.669—1.898	**1.886**	**1.015—3.504**
Index Child Sex (female)	.872	.532—1.427	1.054	.583—1.906
Respondent age (years)	1.006	.962—1.052	.994	.942—1.050
Index Child Age	1.042	.990—1.097	1.035	.974—1.101
Number of children < 5 years	.940	.678—1.304	.918	.619—1.362
Education	1.017	.925—1.119	1.050	.937—1.177
Household Dietary Diversity Score	1.040	.901—1.201	.978	.822—1.162

Note. Bold indicates significance at the .05 level.

Table 20

Results of the Multinomial Logistic Regression for Where Treatment Was Sought for Child Illness

	Where treatment was sought for child illness							
	Community Health Worker vs. Health Center (reference)		Hospital vs. Health Center (reference)		Private Clinic vs. Health Center (reference)		Other vs. Health Center (reference)	
Variable	Odds	95% CI	Odds	95% CI	Odds	95% CI	Odds	95% CI
Probable depression status	.674	.363—1.253	.552	.267—1.140	1.948	.677—5.607	.896	.164—4.901
Head of Household (respondent)	**.245**	**.091—.657**	.352	.091—1.359	.557	.139—2.238	4.325	.862—21.698
Marital status (partnered)	.489	.233—1.025	2.325	.639—8.453	1.028	.340—3.106	4.252	.381—47.402
Employed	1.104	.633—1.927	1.887	.990—3.596	**2.405**	**1.222—4.731**	**3.406**	**1.035—11.209**
Index Child Sex (female)	.621	.381—1.011	**1.840**	**1.024—3.307**	1.545	.808—2.955	.696	.224—2.165
Respondent age (years)	**1.093**	**1.043—1.145**	1.052	.995—1.112	.999	.936—1.066	.952	.858—1.057
Index Child Age	1.022	.971—1.075	1.008	.949—1.070	.942	.881—1.007	.961	.858—1.076
Number of children < 5 years	.889	.642—1.231	1.002	.679—1.477	.757	.487—1.177	.766	.349—1.682
Education	1.022	.931—1.121	1.079	.965—1.206	**1.174**	**1.030—1.340**	.859	.690—1.068
Household Dietary Diversity Score	.899	.782—1.033	.883	.746—1.044	1.001	.836—1.198	**1.372**	**1.031—1.824**

Note. Bold indicates significance at the .05 level.

Table 21

Results of Poisson Regression Analysis for Knowledge of Danger Signs of Childhood Illness

Variable	B	Robust SE	*Wald χ²*	Exp(B)	95% CI for Exp(B)
Probable depression status (Depressed)	1.54	0.07	439.85***	4.65	4.03—5.37
Head of household (respondent)	-0.07	0.06	1.18	0.94	0.83—1.06
Marital status (partnered)	.07	.06	1.63	1.08	0.96—1.21
Employed	-.05	0.04	1.93	0.95	0.89—1.02
Index child sex (female)	-0.04	0.03	1.70	0.96	0.90—1.02
Respondent age (years)	0.01	0.003	4.22*	1.01	1.00—1.01
Index child age	-0.001	0.003	0.12	1.00	0.99—1.01
Number of children < 5 years	-0.02	0.02	1.16	0.98	0.93—1.02
Education	0.01	0.01	3.56	1.01	1.00—1.02
Household dietary diversity score	0.03	0.01	7.33**	1.03	1.01—1.05

Note: N=1280. *p<.05, **p<.01, ***p<.001.

Infant and Young Child Feeding Practices

To examine the bivariate relationships between probable depression status and behaviors in the domain of infant and young child feeding behaviors, chi-square tests of independence and Mann-Whitney U-tests were run. Depressed and nondepressed respondents were found to statistically significantly differ in whether a child was fed the same amount or more food than usual during illness, $\chi^2(1) = 5.86$, $p = .016$, whether a child was offered more fluids than usual during illness, $\chi^2(1) = 12.80$, $p < .001$, whether a child of 6-23 months met criteria for minimum dietary diversity, $\chi^2(1) = 9.19$, $p = .010$, whether a child in this same age group meets criteria for minimum meal frequency, $\chi^2(1) = 12.39$, $p < .001$, whether a child younger than 6 months was exclusively breastfed, $\chi^2(1) = 4.03$, $p = .045$, the number of complementary feedings provided to children 6-23 months in the previous 24-hour period, $U = 49167.0$, $z = -3.11$, $p = .002$, and the number of fortified and nutrient-dense complementary foods provided to the 6-23 month index child in the previous 24-hour period, $U = 54224.5$, $z = -5.93$, $p < .001$ (See table 22).

A series of logistic and hierarchical multiple regressions were then carried out for the variables with statistically significant results to determine differential odds for a given behavior between depressed and nondepressed respondents or the variance accounted for by probable depression status in a continuous outcome variable. Covariates for these analyses included participant age, child age, child sex, number of children under 5 years living in the household, marital status, whether the participant is employed, head of household (respondent or other), respondent's years of education, and household dietary diversity score. The results of the logistic regression run for the amount of drink offered to a child during illness are not presented here due to sparse data bias, which rendered the parameter estimates for these analyses uninterpretable. Further analyses on this outcome variable were therefore unable to be run.

Binomial logistic regressions were run to determine the effects of depression on the likelihood that participants had provided the same or more food than usual to children 6-23 months old, as recommended in the WHO guidelines for infant and young child feeding practices (World Health Organization, 2003).

The final model of the logistic regression predicting likelihood of more food intake during illness was statistically significant, $\chi^2(10) = 18.49$, $p = .047$. The model explained 4.9% (Nagelkerke R^2) of the variance in amount of food offered and correctly classified 83.2% of cases. Probable depression status was a statistically significant predictor of the amount of food offered to a sick child above and beyond the effects of the aforementioned covariates, none of which reached significance in this model (see Table 23). Depressed participants had 2.37 higher odds of offering their child the same amount or more food than usual to their sick child.

A logistic regression was also run to determine the effects of depression on the likelihood that their 6-23-month-old child's food intake in the previous 24-hour period met criteria for minimum dietary diversity. The model was statistically significant, $\chi^2(10) = 68.80$, $p < .001$, and explained 28.3% (Nagelkerke R^2) of the variance in minimum dietary diversity. Depression did not reach significance as a predictor of reaching minimum dietary diversity, however (see Table 23). Statistical significance was also reached for the model ascertaining the effects of probable depression status on the likelihood that their child's frequency of meals in the previous 24-hour period met the WHO IYCF guidelines criteria for minimum meal frequency, $\chi^2(10) = 694.52$, $p < .001$. The model explained 55.4% of the variance in minimum meal frequency (Nagelkerke R^2)

and correctly classified 80.0% of cases. However, introducing probable depression status, $\chi^2(1) =$ 1.31, $p = .253$, did not improve the model's prediction of this outcome variable (see Table 23).

The model of the hierarchical multiple regression ascertaining the effects of depression on the number of complementary feedings followed a similar pattern. While model 1 of this test achieved statistical significance, $R^2 = .066$, $F(9, 776) = 6.12$, $p < .001$; adjusted $R^2 = .055$, the addition of probable depression status in model 2 did not statistically significantly improve the prediction of the number of complementary feedings given to a 6-23 month child in the previous 24 hours, $R^2 = .068$, $F(1, 775) = 1.67$, $p = .193$; adjusted $R^2 = .056$ (See table 24).

For the hierarchical multiple regression predicting the number of fortified and nutrient-dense complementary foods provided for 6-23 month old children in the previous 24 hours, probable depression status did improve the prediction of this outcome. The full model (Model 2) was statistically significant, $R^2 = .256$ $F(1, 877) = 23.771$, $p < .0005$; adjusted $R^2 = .247$. The addition of probable depression status to the prediction of the number of fortified and nutrient-dense complementary foods in the previous 24-hour period (Model 2) led to a statistically significant increase in R^2 of .020. Nondepressed mothers provided their child on average 0.324 more fortified and nutrient-dense complementary foods in the previous 24-hour period than their nondepressed counterparts (See table 25).

Table 22

Summary for Tests of Differences in IYCF Behaviors Between Probably Depressed and Non-Depressed Respondents

| | Depression status | | | | |
| Measure | Probably Depressed (n = 1012) | | Not Depressed (n = 282) | | Test Statistic |
	n	*%*	*n*	*%*	
Same or more food than usual offered to sick child	98	18.8	10	9.2	$\chi^2 = 5.86*$
More fluid than usual offered to sick child	55	9.6	0	0	$\chi^2 = 12.80***$
Exclusive breastfeeding of child <6 months	300	89.3	66	91.7	$\chi^2 = 0.36$
Breastfeeding of child 6-23 months	655	94.4	202	95.3	$\chi^2 = 0.26$
Complementary feeding of child (6-23 mos)	611	88.0	188	88.7	$\chi^2 = 0.06$
Minimum Dietary Diversity	31	3.0	3	1.1	$\chi^2 = 9.19*$
Minimum Meal Frequency	476	46.3	165	58.1	$\chi^2 = 12.39***$
	Mean *(SD)*		**Mean *(SD)***		
Number of complementary feedings in 24 hours	2.29 *(1.11)*		2.57 *(0.99)*		$z = -3.11**$
Number of breast feedings in 24 hours (6-23 mos)	13.01 *(5.82)*		11.89 *(3.55)*		$z = 1.24$
Dietary Diversity (6-23 mos)	2.40 *(1.24)*		2.49 *(1.01)*		$z = -0.30$
Number of fortified and nutrient dense complementary foods provided (6-23 mos)	1.30 *(0.85)*		1.67 *(0.69)*		$z = -5.93***$

Notes. * $p < .05$ (two-tailed). ** $p < .01$ (two-tailed). *** $p < .001$ (two-tailed).

Table 23

Results of Binomial Logistic Regressions for IYCF Behaviors

Variables	Same or more food offered to child during illness	Minimum dietary diversity	Minimum meal frequency
	OR (95% CI)	OR (95% CI)	OR (95% CI)
Probable depression status (Depressed)	2.37 (1.12—5.00)*	4.11 (0.87—19.46)	0.81 (0.54—1.20)
Head of Household (respondent)	0.48 (0.18—1.22)	0.36 (0.07—1.89)	0.58(0.33—1.02)
Marital status (partnered)	0.81 (0.39—1.70)	0.33 (0.11—1.01)	0.77 (0.46—1.28)
Employed	1.06 (0.68—1.67)	1.55 (0.68—3.52)	1.01 (0.73—1.41)
Index Child Sex (female)	1.10 (0.71—1.69)	1.30 (0.59—2.85)	1.15 (0.85—1.55)
Respondent age (years)	1.02 (0.98—1.06)	1.01 (0.95—1.09)	1.02 (0.10—1.05)
Index Child Age	0.96 (0.91—1.00)	1.04 (0.94—1.17)	1.45 (1.40—1.51)***
Number of children < 5 years	0.97 (0.73—1.29)	1.27 (0.75—2.15)	0.98 (0.80—1.20)
Education	0.94 (0.87—1.02)	1.06 (0.92—1.23)	0.98 (0.93—1.04)
Household Dietary Diversity Score	1.07 (0.94—1.21)	2.05 (1.66—2.54)***	1.19 (1.09—1.30)***

Note. N=619, N= 851, N=1294, respectively. *p<.05, **p<.01, ***p<.001.

Table 24

Results of Hierarchical Multiple Regression Analysis for Number of Complementary Feedings in the Previous 24-Hour Period

Variable	Model 1 B	Model 1 β	Model 2 B	Model 2 β
	Number of Complementary Feedings in the Previous 24-hour Period			
Probable depression status			-0.13	-0.05
Head of Household (respondent)	-.09	-.02	-.08	-.02
Marital status (partnered)	0.13	0.04	0.12	0.03
Employed	-0.07	-0.03	-0.03	-0.01
Index Child Sex (female)	0.07	0.03	0.07	0.03
Respondent age (years)	0.01*	0.08	0.01*	0.08
Index Child Age	0.05***	0.16	0.05***	0.15
Number of children < 5 years	-0.06	-0.04	-0.05	-0.03
Education	0.010	.03	0.01	0.03
Household Dietary Diversity Score	0.10***	0.16	0.11***	0.17
R^2	.07		.07	
F	6.12***		5.68***	
ΔR^2	.07		.002	
ΔF	6.12***		1.70	

Note: N=786. *p<.05, **p<.01, ***p<.001

99

Table 25

Results of Hierarchical Multiple Regression Analysis for Provision of Fortified and Nutrient-Dense Complementary Foods Among Children 6-23 months

	Model 1		Model 2	
Variable	B	β	B	β
Probable depression status (Nondepressed)			0.32***	0.16
Head of Household (respondent)	-0.05	-0.02	-0.01	-0.003
Marital status (partnered)	0.001	0.0002	-0.01	-0.01
Employed	-0.09	-0.05	0.01	0.003
Index Child Sex (female)	0.04	0.02	0.05	0.03
Respondent age (years)	-0.01	-0.06	-0.01	-0.05
Index Child Age	0.05***	0.20	0.04***	0.18
Number of children < 5 years	-0.07	-0.06	-0.06	-0.05
Education	-0.01	-0.03	-0.01	-0.03
Household Dietary Diversity Score	0.21***	0.42	0.22***	0.43
R^2	.24		.26	
F	30.06		30.13	
ΔR^2	.24		.02	
ΔF	30.06		23.77	

Note: N=888. *p<.05, **p<.01, ***p<.001.

Water, Sanitation and Hygiene Behaviors

To examine the bivariate relationships between probable depression status and WASH

behaviors, chi-square tests of independence were run. Differences between depressed and

nondepressed respondents were statistically significant for the type of handwashing station in the

household $\chi^2(2) = 25.24$, $p < .001$, where their child under 24 months last defecated, $\chi^2(7) =$

104.42, $p < .001$, the location in which this fecal matter was disposed, $\chi^2(11) = 52.33$, $p < .001$,

and whether household water was treated to make it safe for drinking, $\chi^2(1) = 32.56$, $p < .001$

(see Table 26).

A logistic regression was run for each outcome variable to determine the effects of

probable depression status on its prediction. The model performed to ascertain the effects of

depression on the availability of a soap-and-water handwashing station in the household was

statistically significant, $\chi^2(10) = 79.43$ $p < .001$, explained 8% (Nagelkerke R^2) of the variance in

this variable and correctly classified 61.6% of cases. Probable depression status was found to

significantly improve this model's prediction (see Table 27). Depressed participants were 56%

more likely to have a soap-and-water handwashing station in the home.

The model run to determine the effects of depression on the safe disposal of child feces

was also statistically significant, $\chi^2(10) = 137.83$ $p < .001$, explained 17.3% (Nagelkerke R^2) of

the variance in disposal method of feces and correctly classified 84% of cases. Probable

depression status was found to significantly improve this model's prediction (see Table 27).

Nondepressed participants had 2.5 higher odds (OR=2.51, CI: 1.48, 4.26) of using a safe disposal

method for their child's feces compared to depressed mothers.

Statistical significance was also reached by the model examining the effects of depression

on the use of an adequate water treatment method for household drinking water, $\chi^2(10) = 50.69$,

$p < .001$. The model explained 9.9% (Nagelkerke R^2) of the variance in the use of an adequate

treatment method and correctly classified 93.3% of cases. While use of an adequate treatment

method for household drinking water was overall quite low (6.7%) in this sample, probable

depression status was a statistically significant predictor in the model (see Table 27). Depressed

participants were more than three times as likely (OR=3.35, CI: 1.41, 8.00) to use an adequate

treatment method than their nondepressed counterparts.

Table 26

Summary for Tests of Differences in WASH Behaviors Between Probably Depressed and Non-Depressed Respondents

| | Depression status | | | | |
| | Probably Depressed (n = 1012) | | Not Depressed (n = 282) | | |
Measure	n	%	n	%	Test Statistic
Soap and water handwashing station in household	476	46.3	89	31.3	$\chi^2 = 20.33$***
Child defecation location					$\chi^2 = 104.42$***
In the open within house yard	114	40.1	114	40.1	
Fecal matter disposal location					$\chi^2 = 52.33$***
Dropped into toilet facility	583	66.1	225	80.9	
Safe disposal of child feces	840	81.7	265	93.3	$\chi^2 = 22.53$***
Adequate Drinking Water Treatment	82	8.0	6	2.1	$\chi^2 = 12.23$***

Note. * $p < .05$ (two-tailed). ** $p < .01$ (two-tailed). *** $p < .001$ (two-tailed).

Table 27

Results of Binomial Logistic Regressions for WASH Behaviors

Variables	Soap and water handwashing facility in household	Safe disposal of child feces	Use of adequate water treatment method
	OR (95% CI)	OR (95% CI)	OR (95% CI)
Probable depression status	1.57 (1.15—2.13)**	0.40 (0.24—0.67)**	3.35 (1.41—8.00)**
Head of Household (respondent)	1.15 (0.75—1.74)	1.17 (0.64—2.13)	2.45 (1.21—4.97)*
Marital status (partnered)	0.93 (0.63—1.36)	0.90 (0.51—1.57)	1.93 (0.83—4.49)
Employed	1.90 (1.48—2.44)***	0.78 (0.56—1.09)	1.33 (0.84—2.11)
Index Child Sex (female)	0.77 (0.61—0.96)*	1.14 (0.83—1.57)	0.87 (0.55—1.35)
Respondent age (years)	0.99 (0.97—1.01)	0.98 (0.95—1.01)	0.93 (0.89—0.97)**
Index Child Age	1.01 (0.98—1.03)	1.18 (1.14—1.22)***	0.96 (0.92—1.00)
Number of children < 5 years	1.13 (0.96—1.32)	0.99 (0.80—1.23)	1.09 (0.81—1.47)
Education	1.08 (1.04—1.13)***	1.01 (0.95—1.07)	1.07 (0.98—1.17)
Household Dietary Diversity Score	1.01 (0.95—1.08)	1.01 (0.92—1.11)	1.11 (0.98—1.25)

Note. N=1294. *p<.05, **p<.01, ***p<.001.

Child Illness Prevention Behaviors

To examine the bivariate relationships between probable depression status and child illness prevention behaviors, chi-square tests of independence were run. Differences between depressed and nondepressed respondents were statistically significant for whether the household had an insecticide-treated mosquito net, $\chi^2(1) = 998.70$, $p < .001$, whether the index child slept under this treated net, $\chi^2(1) = 979.25$, $p < .001$, and whether the index child's growth has ever been monitored, $\chi^2(1) = 13.35$, $p < .001$ (See Table 28).

The results of the logistic regressions run using the availability of an insecticide-treated mosquito net in the household and whether the index child slept under this treated net as outcome variables are not presented here due to sparse data bias, which rendered the parameter estimates for these analyses uninterpretable. Further analyses on these outcome variables were therefore unable to be performed.

The results of the logistic regression examining the relationships between probable depression status and the remaining child illness prevention behavior, monitoring of child's growth, are presented in Table 29. The logistic regression model for this outcome variable was statistically significant, $\chi^2(10) = 485.62$, $p < .001$, explained 41.8% (Nagelkerke R^2) of the variance in child growth monitoring, and correctly classified 77.4% of cases. Depression was not a significant predictor in this model, however.

Table 28

Summary for Tests of Differences in Child Illness Prevention Behaviors Probably Between Depressed and Non-Depressed Respondents

| | Depression status | | | | |
| | Probably Depressed (n = 1012) | | Not Depressed (n = 282) | | |
Measure	*n*	*%*	*n*	*%*	Test Statistic
Insecticide-treated mosquito net in household	978	95.1	11	3.9	χ^2 = 998.70***
Child slept under mosquito net	962	93.6	3	1.1	χ^2 = 979.25***
Child growth monitored	526	51.2	180	63.4	χ^2 = 13.35***
Child weight monitored in the last 3 months	52	18.3	185	18.0	χ^2 = 0.02
Receipt of Rotavirus vaccine (6-23 mos.)	339	48.8	91	42.9	χ^2 = 2.29
Vitamin A dose given within last 6 months	228	22.2	52	18.3	χ^2 = 1.98

Notes. Pearson bi-serial correlation

* $p < .05$ (two-tailed). ** $p < .01$ (two-tailed). *** $p < .001$ (two-tailed).

Table 29

Results of Binomial Logistic Regressions for Child Illness Prevention Behaviors

Variables	Index child's growth has been monitored
	OR (95% CI)
Probable depression status	0.78 (0.55—1.12)
Head of Household (respondent)	0.86 (0.52—1.43)
Marital status (partnered)	1.04 (0.65—1.66)
Employed	0.93 (0.69—1.25)
Index Child Sex (female)	0.95 (0.73—1.24)
Respondent age (years)	0.99 (0.92—1.01)
Index Child Age	1.32 (1.28—1.36)***
Number of children < 5 years	0.93 (0.77—1.11)
Education	0.95 (0.91—1.00)
Household Dietary Diversity Score	1.08 (1.00—1.16)

*Note. *p < .05 **p < .005*

Child Health Outcomes

A binomial logistic regression was run to ascertain the effects of probable depression on the likelihood of an index child being underweight, defined by a weight-for-age z-score greater than two standard deviations below the mean. The model was statistically significant, $\chi^2(10) = 22.75$, $p = .012$, explained 7.5% (Nagelkerke R^2) of the variance in this variable and correctly classified 73% of cases. Probable depression status was found to significantly improve the strength of this model (see Table 30). Probably depressed participants were nearly twice as likely (OR=1.977) to have an underweight child than their nondepressed counterparts. The logistic regression model assessing the effects of probable depression on child stunting was insignificant, however, $\chi^2(10) = 11.97$, $p = .287$ (See Table 30).

Table 30

Results of Binomial Logistic Regressions for Child Health Outcomes

Variables	Child underweight	Child stunting
	OR (95% CI)	OR (95% CI)
Probable depression status	1.98 (1.09—3.59)*	0.70 (0.42—1.18)
Head of Household (respondent)	1.26 (0.56—2.86)	1.61 (0.76—3.420
Marital status (partnered)	1.21 (0.57—2.55)	1.04 (0.52—2.08)
Employed	0.73 (0.44—1.21)	1.81 (1.14—2.86)
Index Child Sex (female)	0.86 (0.32—2.31)	1.14 (0.45—2.87)
Respondent age (years	0.99 (0.95—1.03)	1.00 (0.96—1.04)
Index Child Age	1.07 (1.02—1.12)**	1.03 (0.99—1.07)
Number of children < 5 years	1.19 (0.88—1.61)	0.89(0.66—1.19)
Education	0.90 (0.83—0.98)*	0.99 (0.92—1.07)
Household Dietary Diversity Score	1.11 (0.98—1.26)	1.02 (0.91—1.15)

Note. N = 431. *p < .05. **p < .01. ***p < .001.

Aim 3: Examining the Moderating Role of Perceived Social Support

A series of moderation analyses were performed using the SPSS PROCESS Macro to investigate the impact of mothers' perceived social support on (1) the relationship between maternal depression and respondents' demonstration of child health promoting behaviors; (2) the relationship between maternal depression and the prevalence of child underweight (as measured by weight-by-age Z-score); and (3) the relationship between maternal depression and the prevalence of child stunting (as measured by height-by-age Z-score). Covariates included in all analyses in this section were the following: participant age, child age, child sex, number of children under 5 years living in the household, marital status, whether the participant is employed, head of household (respondent or other), respondent's years of education, and household dietary diversity score. MSPSS score was mean-centered to facilitate interpretation of conditional effects.

Child Health Promoting Behaviors

The child health promoting behaviors with which probable depression status was found to have a statistically significant relationship above and beyond the effects of included covariates were entered as outcome variables in a moderated logistic and hierarchical multiple regressions, where probable depression status was the independent variable and mean score for the full MSPSS scale (referred to from here on as MSPSS score) was included as the moderator.

Integrated management of childhood illness (IMCI). Table 31 presents the results of simple moderated logistic regressions with having had a sick child in the last 2 weeks, how long after noticing the child's illness the respondent sought advice or treatment outside the home, and knowledge of at least three danger signs of childhood illness as the outcome variables.

Child illness in the last 2 weeks. The moderation analysis to test whether the interaction between probable depression status and perceived social support (MSPSS score) predicted the probability of having had a child with presumable pneumonia/ARI symptoms was not found significant, $b = 0.283$, 95% C.I. (-0.414, 0.980), $p = .425$.

When advice or treatment was sought for child illness. This interaction was also not significant for the analyses including when care was sought for child illness in the last 2 weeks, $b = 0.037$, 95% C.I. (-0.183, 0.256), $p = .742$.

Knowledge of at least three danger signs of childhood illness. This interaction was also not significant for the analysis including knowledge of at least three danger signs of childhood illness, $b = 0.194$, 95% C.I. (-0.161, 0.548), $p = .283$, as the outcome variable.

Table 31

Moderation Effects of Perceived Social Support (MSPSS) on the Relationship Between Depression Status and IMCI Behaviors

| | Outcome Variable | | | | | | | | |
| | Child illness in last 2 weeks | | | When treatment sought for child illness | | | Knowledge of ≥ 3 danger signs of child illness | | |
Variable	Coefficient	*SE* B	*z*	Coefficient	*SE* B	*z*	Coefficient	*SE* B	*z*
Head of Household (respondent)	-0.33	0.31	-1.08	-0.09	0.15	-0.62	-0.23	0.45	-0.51
Education (yrs.)	0.03	0.03	0.98	0.00	0.01	0.00	0.04	0.04	0.98
Employed	0.11	0.18	0.64	-0.01	0.08	-0.11	-0.09	0.25	-0.35
Household dietary diversity	-0.06	0.05	-1.21	0.00	0.02	0.20	0.13	0.73	1.83
Child sex (Female)	-0.15	0.15	-0.99	0.09	0.07	1.22	0.16	0.55	0.30
Child age (mos.)	-0.01	0.02	-0.51	0.00	0.01	-0.21	0.004	0.23	0.16
Respondent age (yrs.)	-0.01	0.01	-0.45	0.00	0.01	-0.55	0.01	0.21	0.30
Partnered	-0.26	0.30	-0.87	0.09	0.13	0.70	0.56	0.41	1.39
Number of children <5 years	0.05	0.11	0.45	-0.09	0.05	-1.71	0.06	0.16	0.37
Probable depression status	0.34	0.25	1.39	0.12	0.12	0.95	3.64***	0.98	3.70
MSPSS score	-0.44	0.33	-1.33	-0.18	0.17	-1.07	1.11	1.35	0.82
Depression X MSPSS score	0.28	0.36	0.80	0.19	0.18	1.07	-1.69	1.37	-1.24
Model χ^2 *(df)*	19.44*(12)*						91.57*(12)***		
Nagelkerke R^2	0.04						0.29		
F				1.04					
F change				1.15					
R^2				0.03					
R^2 change				0.003					

Note. * $p < .05$. ** $p < .01$. *** $p < .001$.

Infant and young child feeding practices. Table 32 presents the results of a simple moderated

logistic regression with the amount of food fed to a sick child as the outcome variable, and Table

33 outlines the results of a moderated multiple regression, which was run to determine the

moderating role of perceived social support on the relationship between probable depression

status and the number of fortified and nutrient-dense complementary foods provided for the 6-23

month index child in the previous 24-hour period.

Amount of food offered to child during illness. The interaction between probable

depression status and MSPSS score to predict the probability of providing the same or more than

the usual amount of food to a child during illness not found to be statistically significant,

$b = -0.21$, 95% C.I. (-2.227, 1.816), $p = .842$.

Provision of fortified and nutrient-dense complementary foods. For this outcome

variable as well, the interaction between probable depression status and perceived social support

was not statistically significant, $b = 0.056$, 95% C.I. (-0.193, 0.304), $p = .661$.

Table 32

Moderation Effects of Perceived Social Support (MSPSS) on the Relationship Between Depression Status and Amount of Food Offered to Child During Illness

Variable	Coefficient	*SE* B	*z*
Head of Household (respondent)	-0.11	0.69	-0.15
Education (yrs.)	-0.10	0.07	-1.40
Employed	0.37	0.40	0.91
Household dietary diversity	0.21	0.12	1.68
Child sex (Female)	0.26	1.11	0.23
Child age (mos.)	0.00	0.05	0.03
Respondent age (yrs.)	0.01	0.03	0.43
Partnered	-0.48	0.63	-0.77
Number of children <5 years	-0.45	0.28	-1.61
PHQ-9 Score (Depression)	-0.01	0.04	-0.27
MSPSS score	-0.42	0.33	-1.27
Depression X MSPSS score	0.02	0.06	0.38
Model χ^2 *(df)*	11.14*(12)*		
Nagelkerke R²	.09		

Note. * $p < .05$. ** $p < .01$. *** $p < .001$.

Table 33

Moderation Effects of Perceived Social Support (MSPSS) on the Relationship Between Depression Status and Provision of Fortified and Nutrient-Dense Complementary Foods

Variable	Coefficient	SE B	t
Head of Household (respondent)	-0.01	0.11	-0.11
Education (yrs.)	-0.01	0.01	-0.52
Employed	-0.04	0.06	-0.57
Household dietary diversity	0.22***	0.02	13.37
Child sex (Female)	0.05	0.06	0.90
Child age (mos.)	0.05***	0.01	6.12
Respondent age (yrs.)	-0.01	0.01	-.1.67
Partnered	-0.08	0.10	-0.80
Number of children <5 years	-0.03	0.04	-0.77
Probable depression status	-0.25**	0.09	-2.86
MSPSS score	0.09	0.12	0.73
Depression X MSPSS score	0.06	0.13	0.44
F	23.92		
F change	.193		
R^2	.285		
R^2 change	.000		

Note. * $p < .05$. ** $p < .01$. *** $p < .001$.

Water, sanitation and hygiene behaviors. Table 34 presents the results of simple moderated logistic regression with availability of a soap-and-water handwashing station in the household, method for disposal of feces, and water treatment method as the outcome variables.

Availability of a soap-and-water handwashing station. The interaction between probable depression status as the independent variable and MSPSS score as the moderator was also statistically significant, [b = 2.31, 95% C.I. (1.50, 3.13), p < .001. The conditional effect of probable depression status on the availability of a handwashing station in the home showed corresponding results at low and high levels of perceived social support, though not at the average level (see Table 35).

For respondents with low perceived social support (1 SD below the sample mean MSPSS score), b = -1.938, z = -4.14, p < .001, probable depression status and availability of a handwashing station are significantly related, such that depression negatively predicts the odds of having a handwashing station, or, depressed participants with low perceived social support have lower odds of having a handwashing station in the home. For respondents with an average level of perceived social support (scores around the sample mean MSPSS score), b = -1.938, z = -1.49, p = .136, probable depression status and availability of a handwashing station are not significantly related. For respondents with high perceived social support (1 SD above the sample mean MSPSS score), b = 1.156, z = 4.29, p < .001, probable depression status and availability of a handwashing station are significantly related, such that probable depression status positively predicts the odds of having a handwashing station, or, depressed participants with high perceived social support have higher odds of having a handwashing station in the home. These results identify perceived social support as a positive moderator of the relationship between probable depression status and having a soap-and-water handwashing station in the household. This interaction is illustrated in Figure 2.

Safe disposal of child fecal matter. The interaction between probable depression status as the independent variable and MSPSS score as the moderator for the prediction of using a safe method for disposal of child feces was not statistically significant, $b = 0.03$, 95% C.I. (-1.55, 1.606), $p = .973$.

Adequate method of water treatment. The interaction between probable depression status as the independent variable and MSPSS score as the moderator for the prediction of using an adequate method of water treatment was also not statistically significant, $b = -2.085$, 95% C.I. (-5.62, 1.45), $p = .248$.

Table 34

Moderation Effects of Perceived Social Support (MSPSS) on the Relationship Between Depression Status and WASH Behaviors

	Outcome Variable								
	Availability of soap-and-water handwashing station			Safe disposal of child fecal matter			Adequate method of water treatment		
Variable	Coefficient	*SE* B	*z*	Coefficient	*SE* B	*z*	Coefficient	*SE* B	*z*
Head of Household (respondent)	-0.02	0.32	-0.05	-0.41	0.48	-0.85	0.39	0.66	0.59
Education (yrs.)	0.07*	0.03	2.35	0.06	0.05	1.25	0.03	0.06	0.56
Employed	0.57**	0.17	3.26	-0.30	0.29	-1.03	0.58	0.33	1.77
Household dietary diversity	0.02	0.05	0.45	0.03	0.08	0.32	0.22*	0.09	2.41
Child sex (Female)	-0.19	0.16	-1.21	0.04	0.27	0.14	-0.22	0.32	-0.71
Child age (mos.)	0.00	0.02	-0.03	0.12**	0.04	3.09	-0.08	0.05	-1.81
Respondent age (yrs.)	-0.01	0.01	-0.78	-0.01	0.02	-0.23	-0.10**	0.03	-2.98
Partnered	-0.08	0.30	-0.28	-0.70	0.59	-1.19	1.61	1.04	1.55
Number of children <5 years	0.09	0.12	0.77	0.02	0.19	0.08	0.31	0.22	1.38
Depression status	-0.39	0.26	-1.49	-0.60	0.55	-1.09	1.89	1.35	1.40
MSPSS score	-1.86***	0.39	-4.76	0.15	0.77	0.19	2.26	1.78	1.28
Depression X MSPSS score	2.31***	0.42	5.56	0.03	0.81	0.03	-2.09	1.80	-1.16
Model χ^2 *(df)*	73.62*(12)*			23.14*(12)*			42.44*(12)*		
Nagelkerke R²	.13			.07			.15		

Note. * $p < .05$. ** $p < .01$. *** $p < .001$.

Table 35

Conditional Effects of Depression Status on Availability of a Handwashing Station (Perceived Social Support)

Perceived Social Support	β	*p*	95% CI
1 SD below mean	-1.94	.000	-2.86 – -1.02
At the mean	-0.39	.136	-0.91 – 0.12
1 SD above mean	1.16	.000	0.63 – 1.69

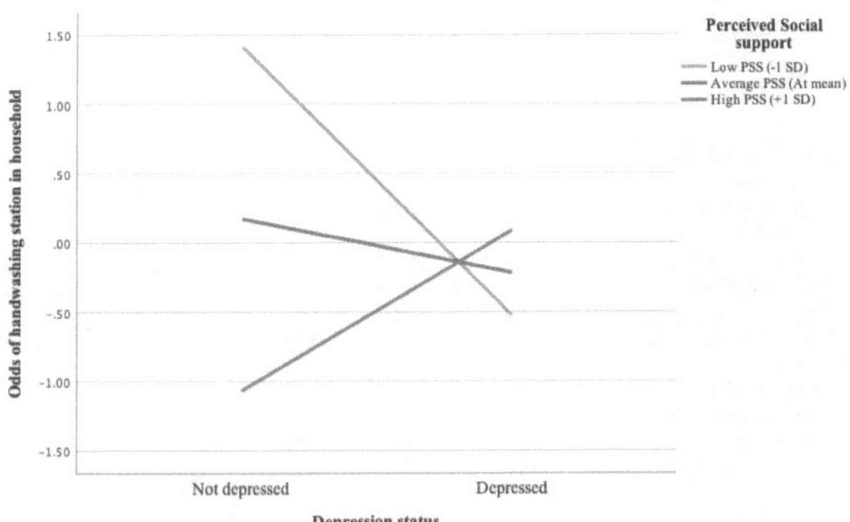

Figure 2: Interaction Between Depression Status and Perceived Social Support for Availability of a Handwashing Station

118

Child health outcomes. Table 36 presents the results of a simple moderated logistic regression with child underweight as the outcome variable.

    Child underweight. The interaction between probable depression status as the independent variable and MSPSS score as the moderator for the prediction of child underweight was not statistically significant, $b = 0.15$, 95% C.I. (-1.10, 1.40), $p = .817$ (See Table 36).

Table 36

Moderation Effects of Perceived Social Support (MSPSS) on the Relationship Between Probable Depression Status and Child Health Outcomes

Parameter	Child Weight-for-Age Z-score (Underweight)		
	Coefficient	*SE* B	*z*
Head of Household (respondent)	0.19	0.48	0.39
Education (yrs.)	-0.08	0.05	-1.81
Employed	-0.30	0.28	-1.08
Household dietary diversity	0.13	0.07	1.81
Child sex (Female)	-0.22	0.56	-0.39
Child age (mos.)	0.07**	0.02	2.92
Respondent age (yrs.)	-0.01	0.02	-0.45
Partnered	0.12	0.43	0.27
Number of children <5 years	0.22	0.17	1.33
Probable depression status	0.62	0.44	1.42
MSPSS score	-0.04	0.60	-0.06
Depression X MSPSS score	0.15	0.64	0.23
Model χ^2 *(df)*	19.72*(12)*		
Nagelkerke R^2	0.08		

Note. * $p < .05$. ** $p < .01$. *** $p < .001$.

Aim 4: Examining the Moderating Role of Women's Empowerment Indicators

A series of moderation analyses were performed using PROCESS to investigate the

impact of women's empowerment indicators (household decision-making, attitudes toward

intimate partner violence, and use of contraception) on (1) the relationship between maternal

depression and respondents' demonstration of child health promoting behaviors; (2) the

relationship between maternal depression and the prevalence of child underweight (as measured

by weight-by-age Z-score); and (3) the relationship between maternal depression and the

prevalence of child stunting (as measured by height-by-age Z-score). Covariates included in all

analyses in this section were the following: participant age, child age, child sex, number of

children under 5 years living in the household, marital status, whether the participant is

employed, head of household (respondent or other), respondent's years of education, and

household dietary diversity score. Moderating variables were mean-centered to facilitate

interpretation of conditional effects.

Operationalization of Household Decision Making

A composite variable was created totaling participant responses to eight household

decision making items taken from the Gender and Family Planning and Birth Spacing modules

of the KPC (Monitoring, C.O.R.E., & Evaluation Working Group, 1999). These included the

following: who has the final say on what to cook, children's healthcare, children's education,

support for the respondent's relatives, support for the relatives of the respondent's partner,

fostering children, children's marriage, and the weight of the respondent's opinion in the

household compared to her male partner. Item responses indicating the participant makes alone

or the participant and her partner jointly make a decision was coded as 1, and item responses indicating the participant's partner alone or a person other than the respondent makes a decision was coded as 0. The household decision making composite variable has a possible range of zero to 8, with higher scores indicating greater decision-making power.

Operationalization of Attitudes toward Intimate Partner Violence

Attitudes toward intimate partner violence were assessed using items taken from the Gender and Family Planning module of the KPC. These items are also represented in the DHS Woman's Questionnaire administered in Uganda. The items ask the respondent whether a male partner is justified in hitting or beating his female partner under six circumstances: if she leaves without telling him, neglects the children, argues with him, refuses sex with him, burns the food, sleeps with another man, or any other reason the respondent feels is justified. The IPV composite variable has a possible range of 0 to 7, with higher scores indicating greater acceptance of IPV.

Operationalization of Use of Contraception

Current use of contraception was assessed using a single item asking the respondent whether she currently uses any method to delay or avoid getting pregnant. Items are coded as 1 if she reports current use of a contraceptive method.

Child health promoting behaviors. The child health promoting behaviors with which probable depression status was found to have a statistically significant relationship above and beyond the effects of included covariates were entered as outcome variables in a series of moderated logistic and moderated hierarchical multiple regressions, where probable depression status was the independent variable and household decision-making, IPV or use of contraception was included as the moderator. These findings are detailed below.

Integrated management of childhood illness (IMCI). The following section details the results of simple moderated logistic regressions with having had a sick child in the last 2 weeks, how long after noticing the child's illness the respondent sought advice or treatment outside the home, and knowledge of at least three danger signs of childhood illness as the outcome variables.

Child illness in the last 2 weeks. The moderation analysis to test whether the interaction between probable depression status and household decision-making predicted the probability of having had a child with presumable pneumonia/ARI symptoms was not found significant, $b = 0.104$, 95% C.I. (-0.039, 0.247), $p = .153$. Statistical significance was also not met for the interaction between probable depression status and attitudes toward IPV, $b = -0.02$, 95% C.I. (-0.185, 0.140), $p = .786$. The interaction between probable depression status and contraception use did achieve significance, however, $b = -0.731$ 95% C.I. (-1.436, -0.027), $p = .042$ (See Table 37). This interaction is illustrated in Figure 3.

Probing of the conditional effects of probable depression status at both levels of contraception use reveals that probable depression status is significantly related to child illness in the last 2 weeks only among women who denied current use of a contraceptive method ($p < .001$). For women in this group only, depressed participants were significantly more likely to have had a child with presumable pneumonia/ARI symptoms in the last two weeks compared to nondepressed women (see Table 38).

When advice or treatment was sought for child illness. Table 39 presents the results of the moderated analyses of WE indicators for when advice of treatment was sought for child illness. Neither the interactions between probable depression status and household decision-making, $b = 0.018$, 95% C.I. (-0.055, 0.092), $p = .620$, nor probable depression status and

122

contraception use, $b = -0.058$, 95% C.I. (-0.395, 0.279), $p = .737$, was significant in the prediction of when advice or treatment was sought for child illness. Statistical significance was achieved for the interaction of probable depression status and attitudes toward IPV, $b = -0.148$, 95% C.I. (-0.235, -0.060), $p = .001$ (See Figure 4). To probe the interaction, conditional effects of probable depression status were tested at three levels of attitudes toward IPV: one standard deviation below the mean, at the mean, and one standard deviation above the mean. Probable depression status was significantly related to when advice or treatment was sought for child illness at low levels of acceptance of IPV (1 SD below the mean), but not among respondents who demonstrate moderate to high levels of justification of IPV (See Table 40).

Results of the Johnson-Neyman technique indicate that the relationship between probable depression status and when treatment was sought for child illness when justification of IPV was .206 or greater standard deviations below the mean.

Knowledge of at least three danger signs of childhood illness. For the moderation analyses including knowledge of at least three danger signs of childhood illness as the outcome variable, none of the interactions between probable depression status and household decision-making, $b = 0.262$, 95% C.I. (-0.235, 0.760), $p = .302$, justification of IPV $b = -0.518$, 95% C.I. (-1.256, 0.220), $p = .169$, and contraception use, $b = -1.003$, 95% C.I. (-3.446, 1.440), $p = .421$, achieved statistical significance (See Table 41).

Table 37

Moderation Effects of Women's Empowerment Indicators on the Relationship Between Depression Status and Child Illness in the Last Two Weeks

	Moderator								
	Household Decision-Making			Attitudes toward IPV			Contraception Use		
Variable	Coefficient	SE	z	Coefficient	SE	z	Coefficient	SE	z
Head of Household (respondent)	-0.15	0.22	-0.70	-0.14	0.21	-0.63	-0.14	-.22	-0.66
Education (yrs.)	-0.01	0.022	-0.21	-0.003	0.02	-0.12	-0.0004	0.02	-0.02
Employed	0.18	0.13	1.35	0.17	0.13	1.33	0.14	0.13	1.09
Household dietary diversity	-0.01	0.03	-0.35	-0.02	0.03	-0.56	-0.02	0.03	-0.62
Child sex (Female)	-0.12	0.12	-1.05	-0.13	0.12	-1.15	-0.13	0.11	-1.13
Child age (mos.)	0.04	0.01	4.00	0.05***	0.01	4.07	0.04***	0.01	3.86
Respondent age (yrs.)	-0.01	0.01	-1.17	-0.01	0.01	-1.39	-0.01	0.01	-1.26
Partnered	0.08	0.20	0.39	0.05	0.20	0.24	0.02	0.20	0.09
Number of children <5 years	0.09	0.08	1.11	0.11	0.08	1.34	0.11	0.08	1.36
Depression status	0.55	0.16	3.55	0.59***	0.16	3.62	0.71***	0.17	4.22
Moderator	-0.09	0.07	-1.35	-0.004	0.07	-0.06	0.79*	0.33	2.36
Depression X Moderator	0.10	0.07	1.43	-0.02	0.09	-0.27	-0.73*	0.36	-2.03
Model χ² (df)	41.14 (12)***			39.29 (12)***			44.67 (12)***		
Nagelkerke R²	0.043			0.04			.05		

Note. * p < .05. ** p < .01. *** p < .001.

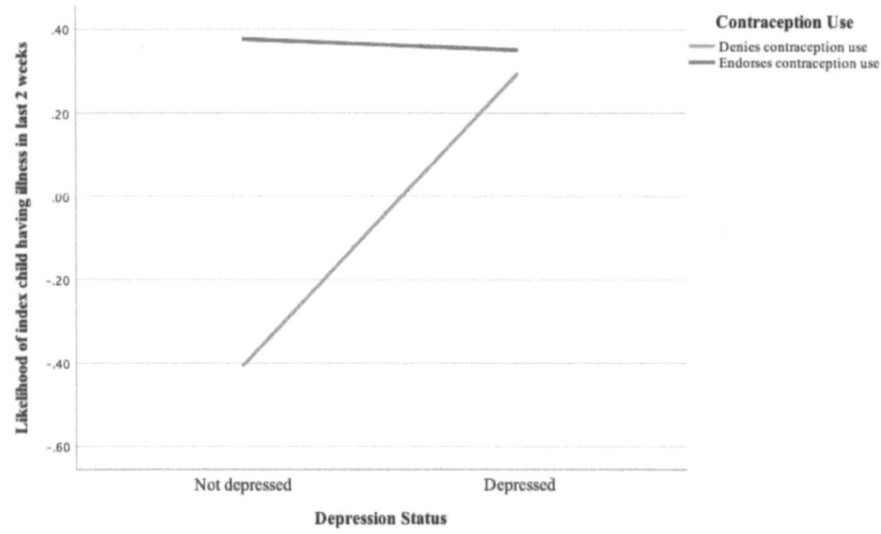

Figure 3: Interaction Between Depression Status and Contraception Use for Child Illness in the Last Two Weeks

Table 38

Conditional Effects of Depression Status on Child Illness in the Last Two Weeks

Use of Contraceptive Method	β	p	95% CI	
No use of contraception	0.71	<.001	0.38	1.03
Use of a contraceptive method	-0.03	.937	-0.67	0.61

125

Table 39

Moderation Effects of Women's Empowerment Indicators on the Relationship Between Depression Status and When Advice or Treatment Was Sought for Child Illness

	Moderator								
	Household Decision-Making			Attitudes toward IPV			Contraception Use		
Variable	Coefficient	SE	t	Coefficient	SE	t	Coefficient	SE	t
Head of Household (respondent)	0.04	0.11	0.40	0.008	0.11	0.08	0.02	0.11	0.21
Education (yrs.)	0.002	0.01	0.22	0.000003	0.01	-0.04	0.000003	0.01	0.0003
Employed	-0.001	0.06	-0.01	0.06	0.06	0.92	0.02	0.06	0.40
Household dietary diversity	-0.01	0.02	-0.76	-0.01	0.02	-0.40	-0.01	0.02	-0.78
Child sex (Female)	0.05	0.06	0.82	0.05	0.06	0.90	0.04	0.06	0.79
Child age (mos.)	-0.01	-0.01	-1.27	-0.01	0.01	-1.50	-0.01	0.01	-1.56
Respondent age (yrs.)	-0.00009	0.01	-0.02	-0.002	0.01	-0.44	-0.002	0.01	-0.35
Partnered	0.16	0.10	1.68	0.14	0.09	1.43	0.14	0.10	1.49
Number of children <5 years	-0.006	0.04	-0.16	0.01	0.04	0.32	0.01	0.04	0.25
Depression status	0.21*	0.08	2.59	0.13	0.09	1.53	0.24	0.09	2.66
Moderator	-0.05	0.03	-1.42	0.10*	0.04	2.43	0.12	0.16	0.77
Depression X Moderator	0.02	0.04	0.50	-0.15**	0.05	-3.32	-0.06	0.17	-0.34
F (df)	1.76 *(12, 609)*			2.69 *12, 619)**￼*			1.67 *(12, 619)*		
F change	0.25 *(1, 609)*			11.00 *(1, 619)**￼*			0.11		
R^2	0.03			.05			0.03		
R^2 change	0.0004			.02			.000		

Note. * $p < .05$. ** $p < .01$. *** $p < .001$.

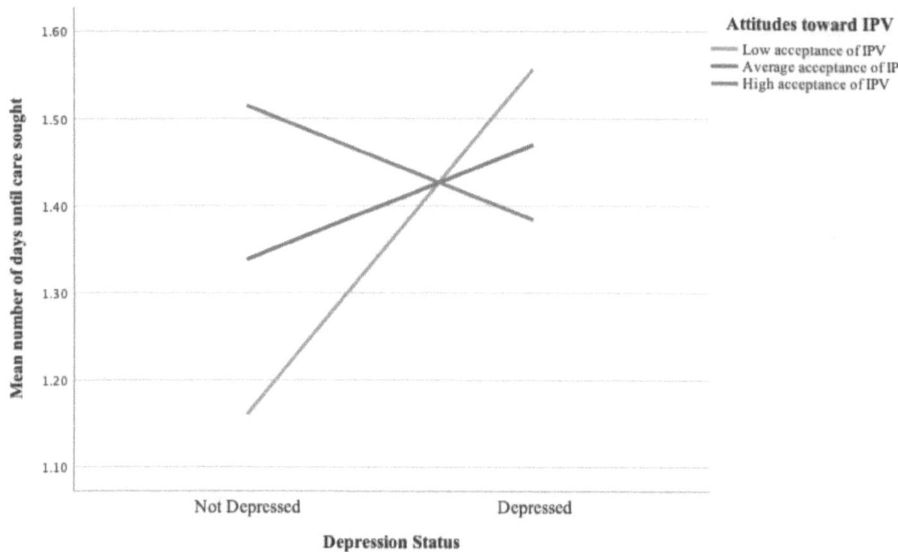

Figure 4: Interaction Between Depression Status and Attitudes Toward IPV on When Advice or Treatment Was Sought for Child Illness

Table 40

Conditional Effects of Depression Status on When Treatment Was Sought for Child Illness

Justification of IPV	β	p	95% CI	
1 SD below mean	0.396	< .001	0.220	0.573
At the mean	0.133	.126	-0.037	0.303
1 SD above mean	-0.131	.349	-0.406	0.144

Table 41

Moderation Effects of Women's Empowerment Indicators on the Relationship Between Depression Status and Knowledge of at Least Three Danger Signs of Childhood Illness

	Moderator								
	Household Decision-Making			Attitudes toward IPV			Contraception Use		
Variable	Coefficient	SE	z	Coefficient	SE	z	Coefficient	SE	z
Head of Household (respondent)	0.06	0.41	0.15	-0.03	0.40	-0.07	0.03	0.39	0.07
Education (yrs.)	0.001	0.04	0.02	-0.001	0.04	-0.02	0.004	0.04	0.12
Employed	-0.14	0.24	-0.60	-0.16	0.24	-0.67	-0.17	0.24	-0.73
Household dietary diversity	1.27	0.07	0.15	0.11	0.07	1.65	0.12	0.07	1.63
Child sex (Female)	0.19	0.50	0.38	0.15	0.50	0.29	0.19	0.50	0.38
Child age (mos.)	-0.002	0.02	-0.08	-0.0004	0.02	-0.02	-0.002	0.02	-0.10
Respondent age (yrs.)	0.01	0.02	0.52	0.01	0.02	0.47	0.01	0.02	0.57
Partnered	0.12	0.37	0.32	0.06	0.36	0.18	0.54	0.35	0.15
Number of children <5 years	0.08	0.15	0.54	0.13	0.15	0.83	0.12	0.15	0.81
Depression status	3.53***	0.59	5.98	3.23***	0.50	6.46	3.36	0.55	6.14
Moderator	0.17	0.29	0.60	0.25	0.27	0.91	0.22	1.16	0.19
Depression X Moderator	-0.25	0.30	-0.85	-0.31	0.28	-1.09	0.03	1.18	0.24
Model χ^2 *(df)*	112.99*(12)* ***			114.08 *(12)****			113.62 *(12)****		
Nagelkerke R²	0.32			0.31			0.31		

Note. * $p < .05.$ ** $p < .01.$ *** $p < .001.$

Infant and young child feeding practices. Tables 42-43 present the results of a simple

moderated logistic regression with the amount of food fed to a sick child as the outcome

variable, and Table 44 outlines the results of a moderated multiple regression, which was run to

determine the moderating role of household decision-making on the relationship between

probable depression status and the number of fortified and nutrient-dense complementary foods

provided for the 6-23 month index child in the previous 24-hour period.

Amount of food offered to child during illness. The moderation analysis to test whether

the interaction between probable depression status and household decision-making to predict the

probability of having fed a sick child the same amount or more food than usual was not found

significant, $b = -0.165$, 95% C.I. (-0.577, 0.246), $p = .431$. The interaction between probable

depression status and justification of IPV, $b = -0.02$, 95% C.I. (-0.185, 0.140), $p = .786$, also

failed to reach statistical significance.

The interaction between probable depression status and contraception use was

statistically significant, $b = -1.787$, 95% C.I. (-3.282, -0.291), $p = .019$. This interaction is

illustrated in Figure 5. Probing of the conditional effects of probable depression status at both

levels of contraception use reveals that probable depression status is significantly related to the

amount of food offered a sick child among women who denied current use of a contraceptive

method ($p = .006$). For women in this group only, depressed participants were significantly

more likely to have fed their child the same or more food than usual while ill, per WHO IYCF

guidelines (see Table 43).

Provision of fortified and nutrient-dense complementary foods. For the moderation

analyses including the number of fortified and nutrient-dense complementary foods provided in

the previous 24 hours for the index child as the outcome variable, none of the interactions

between probable depression status and household decision-making, $b = 0.025$, 95% C.I. (-0.037,

0.087), $p = .426$, justification of IPV $b = 0.025$, 95% C.I. (-0.037, 0.087), $p = .426$, and

contraception use, $b = 0.225$, 95% C.I. (-0.516, 0.066), $p = .129$, achieved statistical significance

(See Table 44).

Table 42

Moderation Effects of Women's Empowerment Indicators on the Relationship Between Depression Status and Amount of Food Offered to Child During Illness

	Moderator								
	Household Decision-Making			Attitudes toward IPV			Contraception Use		
Variable	Coefficient	SE	z	Coefficient	SE	z	Coefficient	SE	z
Head of Household (respondent)	-0.75	0.49	-1.53	-0.75	0.48	-1.56	-0.77	0.49	-1.59
Education (yrs.)	-0.06	0.04	-1.49	-0.06	0.04	-1.41	-0.06	0.04	-1.44
Employed	0.09	0.23	0.37	0.07	0.23	0.32	0.06	0.23	0.24
Household dietary diversity	0.05	0.07	0.79	0.08	0.07	1.18	0.07	0.06	1.10
Child sex (Female)	0.06	0.22	0.26	0.11	0.22	0.49	0.10	0.22	0.44
Child age (mos.)	-0.04	0.02	-1.82	-0.04	0.02	-1.87	-0.05*	0.02	-1.99
Respondent age (yrs.)	0.01	0.02	0.63	0.02	00.02	0.85	0.02	0.02	0.94
Partnered	-0.32	0.39	-0.83	-0.24	0.38	-0.63	-0.27	0.38	-0.70
Number of children <5 years	-0.05	0.15	-0.31	-0.03	0.15	-0.20	-0.02	0.15	-0.15
Depression status	0.97*	0.43	2.23	0.68	0.39	1.73	1.49	0.54	2.74
Moderator	0.19	0.20	0.93	0.25	0.21	1.18	1.79*	0.73	2.47
Depression X Moderator	-0.17	0.21	-0.79	-0.29	0.22	-1.30	-1.79*	0.76	-2.34
Model χ^2 (df)	18..05 (12)			20.19 (12)			24.41 (12)*		
Nagelkerke R^2	0.05			.05			.07		

Note. * $p < .05$. ** $p < .01$. *** $p < .001$.

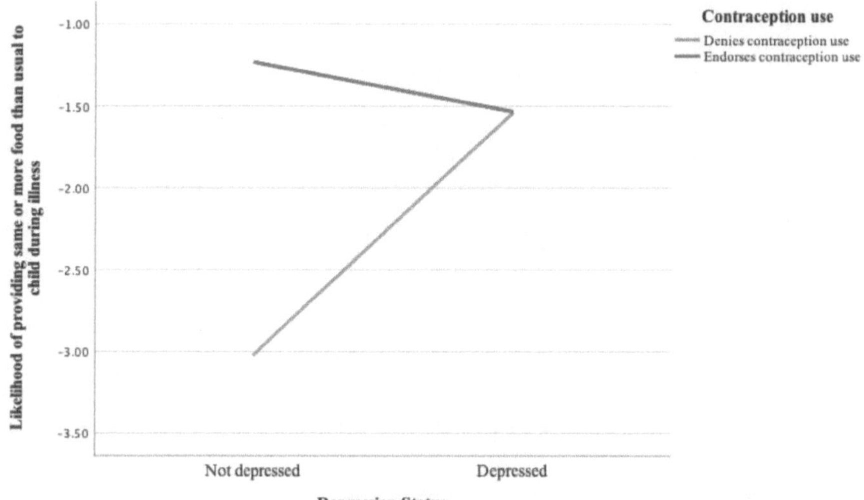

Figure 5: Interaction Between Depression Status and Contraception Use onAamount of Food Offered to Child During Illness

Table 43

Conditional Effects of Depression Status on Amount of Food Offered to Child During Illness

Use of Contraceptive Method	β	*p*	95% CI	
No use of contraception	1.49	.006	0.42	2.55
Use of a contraceptive method	-0.30	.588	-1.39	0.79

Table 44

Moderation Effects of Women's Empowerment Indicators on the Relationship Between Depression Status and Provision of Fortified and Nutrient-Dense Complementary Foods

| | Moderator | | | | | | | | |
| | Household Decision-Making | | | Attitudes toward IPV | | | Contraception Use | | |
Variable	Coefficient	SE	t	Coefficient	SE	t	Coefficient	SE	t
Head of Household (respondent)	-0.01	0.10	-0.11	-0.01	0.10	-0.12	-0.01	0.10	-0.12
Education (yrs.)	-0.01	0.01	-1.02	-0.01	0.01	-1.00	-0.01	0.01	-1.00
Employed	0.002	0.06	0.04	0.0003	0.06	0.004	0.0003	0.06	0.004
Household dietary diversity	0.22***	0.02	14.48	0.21	0.15	14.49	0.21***	0.02	14.48
Child sex (Female)	0.04	0.05	0.81	0.05	0.05	0.91	0.05	0.05	0.95
Child age (mos.)	0.04***	0.01	5.69	0.04	0.01	5.89	0.04***	0.01	5.81
Respondent age (yrs.)	-0.01	0.004	-1.69	-0.01	0.004	-1.62	-0.01	0.004	-1.50
Partnered	-0.04	0.10	-0.48	-0.01	0.09	-0.15	-0.03	0.09	-0.33
Number of children <5 years	-0.06	0.04	-1.50	-0.06	0.04	-1.54	-0.05	0.04	-1.47
Depression status	-0.34***	0.07	-4.93	-0.33	0.07	-4.53	-0.29***	0.08	-3.82
Moderator	-0.01	0.03	-0.24	0.01	0.03	0.15	0.27*	0.14	1.97
Depression X Moderator	0.025	0.03	0.80	-0.01	0.04	-0.15	-0.23	0.15	-1.52
F	25.02 (12, 863)***			25.05 (12, 875)***			25.54 (12, 875)***		
F change	0.64			0.02			2.30		
R^2	.26			.26			.26		
R^2 change	.001			.00002			.005		

Note. * $p < .05$. ** $p < .01$. *** $p < .001$.

Water, sanitation and hygiene behaviors. Tables 45 – 49 present the results of simple

moderated logistic regression with availability of a soap-and-water handwashing station in the

household, method for disposal of feces, and water treatment method as the outcome variables.

Availability of a soap-and-water handwashing station. The interaction between probable

depression status as the independent variable and household decision-making score as the

moderator did not reach statistical significance at the .05 level, $b = 0.134$, 95% C.I. (-0.013,

0.281), $p = .074$. Significant interactions were found for the other two moderating variables,

however (See Table 45). The conditional effects of the significant interaction between probable

depression status and justification of IPV, $b =$ - 0.312, 95% C.I. (-0.495, -0.130), $p = .001$,

indicate a significant relationship between depression and availability of a soap-and-water

handwashing station in the household only at the low level (1 SD below mean) of justification of

IPV (See Figure 6). That is, depressed women are significantly more likely to have a

handwashing station in the home only among women who demonstrate low acceptance of IPV (p

< .001). At moderate and high levels of IPV acceptance, no statistically significant difference

exists between depressed and nondepressed women for this outcome (See Table 46). This

interaction is illustrated in Figure 6. For contraception use, significance was reached only for the

group denying use of a contraceptive method (< .001). As shown in Figure 7, depressed women

who do not use contraception are more likely to have a handwashing station in the household

(See Table 47).

Safe disposal of child fecal matter. The interaction between probable depression status

and household decision-making score also did not reach statistical significance in the prediction of a participant's use of a safe method for disposal of child feces, $b = 0.073$, 95% C.I. (-0.609, 0.600), $p = .989$. For depression and justification of IPV, $b = -0.085$, 95% C.I. (-0.396, 0.226), $p = .592$, and depression and contraception use as well, $b = 0.541$, 95% C.I. (-1.930, 0.463), $p = .230$, these interactions did not reach statistical significance (See Table 48).

Adequate method of water treatment. For this outcome variable as well, none of the interaction variables for the WE moderator variables achieved statistical significance (See table 49).

Table 45

Moderation Effects of Women's Empowerment Indicators on the Relationship Between Depression Status and Availability of a Soap-and-Water Handwashing Station in the Household

	Moderator								
	Household Decision-Making			Attitudes toward IPV			Contraception Use		
Variable	Coefficient	SE	z	Coefficient	SE	z	Coefficient	SE	z
Head of Household (respondent)	0.13	0.22	0.57	0.14	0.22	0.67	0.12	0.22	0.57
Education (yrs.)	0.09***	0.02	3.82	0.08	0.02	3.64	0.08***	0.02	3.55
Employed	0.64***	0.13	4.93	0.60***	0.13	4.68	0.62***	0.13	4.85
Household dietary diversity	0.02	0.03	0.60	0.02	0.03	0.59	0.01	0.03	0.32
Child sex (Female)	-0.28*	0.12	-2.35	-0.23	0.19	-1.96	-0.27	0.12	-2.33
Child age (mos.)	0.01	0.01	0.46	0.01	0.01	0.46	0.003	0.01	0.24
Respondent age (yrs.)	-0.01	0.01	-0.58	-0.01	0.001	-0.69	-0.01	0.01	-0.88
Partnered	-0.06	0.21	-0.28	-0.09	0.20	-0.45	-0.12	0.20	-0.59
Number of children <5 years	0.12	0.08	1.52	0.12	0.08	1.53	0.12	0.08	1.53
Depression status	0.37*	0.16	2.31	0.16	0.17	0.91	0.63***	0.18	3.54
Moderator	-0.13*	0.07	-2.01	0.38***	0.09	4.50	1.01**	0.33	3.04
Depression X Moderator	0.13	0.08	1.78	-0.31**	0.09	-3.35	-0.98**	0.36	-2.71
Model χ^2 (df)	84.86 (12)***			104.87 (12)***			88.60 (12)***		
Nagelkerke R^2	0.09			.11			.09		

Note. * $p < .05$. ** $p < .01$. *** $p < .001$.

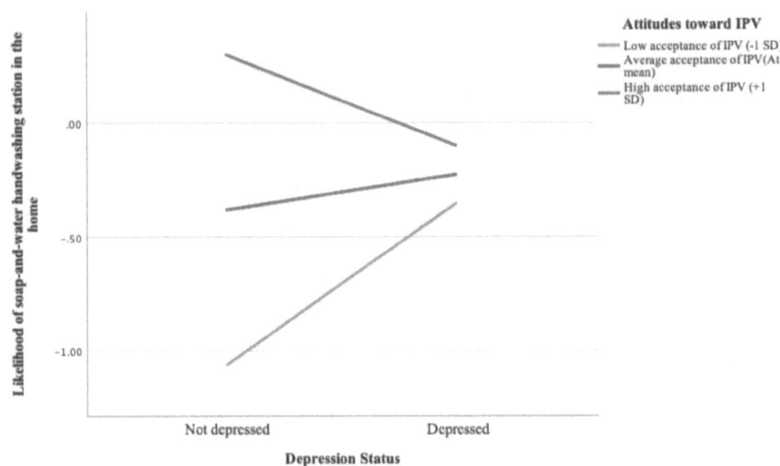

Figure 6: Interaction of Depression Status and Attitudes Toward IPV on Availability of a Soap-and-Water Handwashing Station in the Household

Table 46

Conditional Effects of Depression Status on Availability of a Handwashing Station in the Household (Justification of IPV)

Justification of IPV	β	p	95% CI	
1 SD below mean	0.71	.000	0.32	1.11
At the mean	0.16	.361	-0.18	0.49
1 SD above mean	-0.40	.132	-0.93	0.12

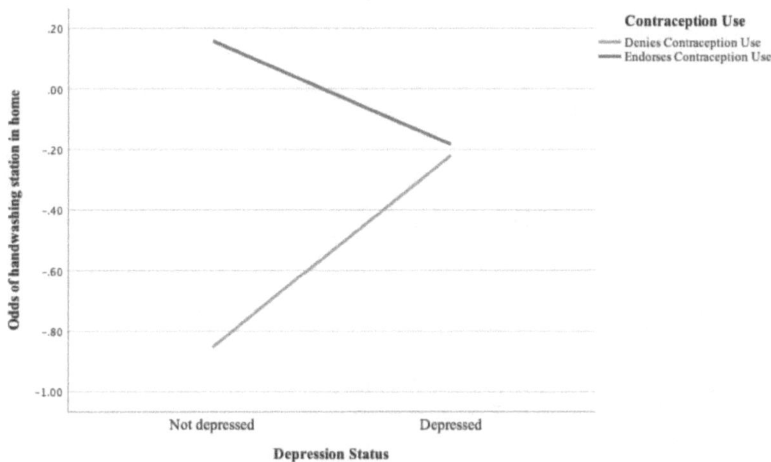

Figure 7: Interaction of Depression Status and Contraception Use on Availability of a Soap-and-Water Handwashing Station in the Household

Table 47

Conditional Effects of Depression Status on Availability of a Handwashing Station in the Household (Use of Contraceptive Method)

Use of Contraceptive Method	β	*p*	95% CI	
No use of contraception	0.63	< .001	0.28	0.99
Use of a contraceptive method	-0.34	.286	-0.97	0.29

Table 48

Moderation Effects of Women's Empowerment Indicators on the Relationship Between Depression Status and Safe Disposal of Child Feces

	Moderator								
	Household Decision-Making			Attitudes toward IPV			Contraception Use		
Variable	Coefficient	*SE*	*z*	Coefficient	*SE*	*z*	Coefficient	*SE*	*z*
Head of Household (respondent)	-0.004	0.31	-0.01	0.14	0.31	0.44	0.14	0.31	0.47
Education (yrs.)	0.01	0.03	0.16	0.001	0.03	0.02	0.01	0.03	0.17
Employed	-0.22	0.17	-1.29	-0.22	0.17	-1.28	-0.22	0.17	-1.30
Household dietary diversity	0.02	0.05	0.32	0.02	0.05	0.33	0.01	0.05	0.15
Child sex (Female)	0.13	0.16	0.77	0.13	0.16	0.81	0.14	0.16	0.86
Child age (mos.)	0.17***	0.02	9.46	0.17***	0.02	9.50	0.17***	0.02	9.56
Respondent age (yrs.)	-0.02	0.01	-1.57	-0.02	0.01	-1.49	-0.02	0.01	-1.45
Partnered	-0.17	0.29	-0.59	-0.133	0.29	-0.44	-0.08	0.29	-0.27
Number of children <5 years	0.002	0.17	0.02	-0.01	0.11	-0.05	-0.02	0.12	-0.15
Depression status	-0.85**	0.28	-3.04	-0.93**	0.31	-3.04	-0.99**	0.30	-3.28
Moderator	0.05	0.13	0.41	0.02	0.15	0.14	-0.73	0.61	-1.20
Depression X Moderator	0.07	0.13	0.55	-0.09	0.16	-0.54	0.54	0.64	0.85
Model χ^2 *(df)*	142.37 (12)***			139.46 (12)***			140.08 (12)***		
Nagelkerke R^2	0.18			.18			0.18		

Note. * $p < .05$. ** $p < .01$. *** $p < .001$.

Table 49

Moderation Effects of Women's Empowerment Indicators on the Relationship Between Depression Status and Use of an Adequate Method of Water Treatment

	Moderator								
	Household Decision-Making			Attitudes toward IPV			Contraception Use		
Variable	Coefficient	SE	z	Coefficient	SE	z	Coefficient	SE	z
Head of Household (respondent)	0.92*	0.37	2.47	0.99*	0.36	2.51	0.90*	0.36	2.49
Education (yrs.)	0.08	0.05	1.70	0.07	0.05	1.51	0.07	0.05	1.49
Employed	0.31	0.24	1.28	0.27	0.24	1.16	0.27	0.24	1.14
Household dietary diversity	0.13*	0.06	2.09	0.10	0.06	1.61	0.10	0.06	1.63
Child sex (Female)	-0.23	0.23	-0.98	-0.13	0.29	-0.57	-0.15	0.23	-0.66
Child age (mos.)	-0.04	0.02	-1.71	-0.04	0.02	-1.79	-0.04	0.02	-1.90
Respondent age (yrs.)	-0.07**	0.02	-3.11	-0.08**	0.02	-3.34	-0.08	0.02	-3.35
Partnered	0.99*	0.50	1.98	0.67	0.43	11.54	0.62	0.43	1.44
Number of children <5 years	0.12	0.16	0.74	0.09	0.15	0.58	0.09	0.15	0.59
Depression status	1.17*	0.47	2.48	1.06*	0.45	2.35	1.39*	0.54	2.58
Moderator	-0.33	0.18	-1.86	0.24	0.24	1.00	0.93	0.89	1.05
Depression X Moderator	0.33	0.19	1.78	-0.21	0.25	-0.84	-0.79	0.92	-0.86
Model χ² (df)	55.64 (12)***			51.86 (12)***			51.93 (12)***		
Nagelkerke R²	0.11			.10			.10		

Note. * $p < .05$. ** $p < .01$. *** $p < .001$.

Child Health Outcomes. Table 50 presents the results of simple moderated logistic regressions including child underweight as the outcome variable.

Child Underweight. As shown in Table 50, the logistic regression models run to determine the moderating effects of each WE indicator on the relationship between probable depression status and the prevalence of child underweight were all statistically significant; however, none of the interaction effects for these analyses achieved statistical significance.

Table 50

Moderation Effects of Women's Empowerment Indicators on the Relationship Between Depression Status and the Incidence of Child Underweight

	Moderator								
	Household Decision-Making			Attitudes toward IPV			Contraception Use		
Variable	Coefficient	SE	z	Coefficient	SE	z	Coefficient	SE	z
Head of Household (respondent)	0.20	0.43	0.45	0.27	0.42	0.65	0.26	0.42	0.63
Education (yrs.)	-0.10*	0.04	-2.32	-0.10*	0.04	-2.34	-0.10*	0.04	-2.46
Employed	-0.37	0.26	-1.42	-0.32	0.26	-1.23	-0.29	0.26	-1.12
Household dietary diversity	0.12	0.07	1.82	0.10	0.07	1.51	0.11	0.07	1.70
Child sex (Female)	-0.16	0.51	-0.32	-0.14	0.51	-0.28	-0.14	0.51	-0.28
Child age (mos.)	0.07	0.02	3.17	0.07**	0.02	2.87	0.06**	0.02	2.70
Respondent age (yrs.)	-0.01	0.02	-0.65	-0.01	0.02	-0.54	-0.01	0.02	-0.55
Partnered	0.12	0.40	0.30	0.20	0.38	0.54	0.20	0.38	0.52
Number of children <5 years	0.16	0.16	1.00	0.16	0.16	1.04	0.17	0.15	1.099
Depression status	0.67*	0.31	2.18	0.85*	0.37	2.31	0.42	0.33	1.27
Moderator	-0.14	0.12	-1.15	-0.16	0.16	-0.98	-1.60	1.08	-1.49
Depression X Moderator	0.21	0.14	1.53	0.21	0.18	1.20	1.82	1.11	1.65
Model χ^2 *(df)*	26.22 (12)**			24.27 (12)*			26.29 (12)**		
Nagelkerke R²	.09			0.08			0.09		

Note. * $p < .05$. ** $p < .01$. *** $p < .001$.

CHAPTER V

DISCUSSION

The purpose of the current study was to explore in a sample of Ugandan mothers of children less than 24 months of age how maternal behaviors affecting child health differed in the presence or absence of maternal depression and to explore how perceived social support and women's empowerment moderated the relationship between maternal depression and mothers' endorsement of these behaviors. This study addressed the gaps in the literature through clarifying the relationships between maternal depression and specific maternal behaviors known to promote child health. This chapter summarizes and contextualizes the study's findings in the extant literature, delineates its limitations and presents directions for further research.

Summary of Findings

Sociodemographic Characteristics

Probably depressed and nondepressed mothers were comparable in most sociodemographic variables, including literacy level, religion, languages spoken, years of education, and household dietary diversity score, which served as a proxy for socioeconomic status in this study, as HDD has been shown to correlate with socioeconomic status and household food security (Hoddinot & Yohannes, 2002; Hatloy, Hallund, Diarra, & Oshaug, 2000; Swindale & Bilinsky, 2006). For both groups, the majority of mothers were at least

143

partially literate, Catholic, Luo-speaking, and non-pregnant. Mothers in both groups also averaged the same number of years of education completed and household dietary diversity.

Unexpectedly, however, substantial differences were found between probably depressed and nondepressed women in employment status, where nondepressed women endorsed earning income outside their home at a much lower rate than their probably depressed counterparts. This finding is in conflict with the current literature examining the relationship between depression and work status, which is most often studied in the context of positive HIV status in Uganda (Wagner et al., 2012; Wagner et al., 2017; Muhwezi et al., 2008). In a 2012 cross-sectional study of this relationship, Wagner and colleagues found that various measures of depression (i.e., PHQ-9 total score, major depression diagnosis) did not remain significantly associated with having worked in the last 7 days after controlling for demographic variables like age, location and education within a sample of Ugandan people living with HIV (Wagner et al., 2012).

Years later, this same research group implemented a prospective randomized controlled trial exploring the relationship between depression alleviation and work productivity, the findings of which indicated that as depressive severity declines the average number of hours worked per week increases (Wagner et al., 2017). The direction of the association between depression and work status established by Wagner and associates served to support the findings of Muhwezi and colleagues, whose study indicated that participants currently experiencing a major depressive episode reported significantly more work-related problems than their nondepressed counterparts (Muhwezi, Agren, Neema, Koma Maganda, & Musisi, 2008).

The current study's finding of probably depressed participants working at higher rates than nondepressed women is of particular interest when considering that no significant

144

differences were found in household socioeconomic status, as measured by household dietary diversity. Given that nondepressed women reported living with a partner at a significantly higher rate and differences were found across the percentages of probably depressed and nondepressed women sampled from each of the six sub-counties covered in this study, it is plausible to conclude that the profound differences in employment status may be partially attributable to differences in permissions and necessity to work as well as work availability.

Seasonality is another imperative variable to consider when examining this unusual difference between groups in work status. As briefly discussed in the methods chapter, a limitation to the current study is the nonconcurrent data collection of probably depressed and nondepressed participants. Because interviewing of probably depressed participants took place from September to early November 2017 while nondepressed participants were interviewed from mid-November to December of that year, how the rainy and dry seasons map onto these interview rounds, and the impact of the seasons on work availability requires acknowledgement.

In Uganda, there are two rainy seasons, and two dry seasons per year; the first interview round of probably depressed participants overlapped with the second rainy season of the year from September to November, and the second interview round of nondepressed participants overlapped with the first dry season, from December to February (Mubangizi, Kyazze, & Mukwaya; 2017). As Kijima, Matsumato and Yamano (2006) note, agricultural production is the primary income source in rural areas of Uganda, and the second cropping season begins in September. As a result, whether a participant earned income outside of her home is more likely attributable to the season during which she was interviewed than her depression status.

Marital status was an additional demographic in which differences were found between probably depressed and nondepressed mothers. Consistent with the extant literature, a higher percentage of nondepressed women described their relationship status as married or living with a partner (Roberts, Ocaka, Browne, Oyok, & Sondorp, 2008; Kakyo, Muliira, Mbalinda, Kizza, & Muliira, 2012). The slight differences found between probably depressed and nondepressed women, where probably depressed women were about 1 year older on average, may bear some relevance to the differences found in relationship status. The head local supervisor for the parent project, which has provided the data for the current study, informed of a cultural practice not addressed in the literature:

> We practice what is called a trial marriage. A woman is brought to be tested on whether she can produce, whether she can work in the garden, her home management skills. That one is so intense where if you don't make it to the satisfaction of the family, chances are high your dowry will not be paid… After two years, the man will go to his parents and sit down and decide about whether they can go ahead and marry. If a man decides to marry a woman, then the man has to pay a price—like a bull—for the children. If the man decides not to marry, this woman goes back to her parents' home with the kids. (A. Akidi, personal communication, August 26, 2020)

This description of trial marriage is of explanatory value to the relationships found between depression, older age and single or divorced relationship status. While directionality cannot be determined (depressive symptoms may be the precipitant, the product, or both, of the dissolution of the trial marriage), it is plausible that participating in a trial marriage and leaving it unmarried would result in being of older age and not partnered. Additionally, the finding that both probably depressed and nondepressed women in this study had a median of two biological children, the chances of remarrying for these depressed women grows slimmer, as De Walque and Kline (2012) point out that women with children are often seen as a liability by men considering marriage. It follows, then, that depressed women, who reported living with a partner at lower rates, would endorse higher rates of heading their households.

Differences in average age of the index child between groups of about 2 months is attributable to the aforementioned methodological limitation of nonconcurrent data collection for the probably depressed and nondepressed groups. Similarly, methodology explains the significant differences found in sub-county residence for these two groups. Due to the convenience sampling procedure employed for the second round of interviewing because of geographical limitations, representation across the six sub-counties included in this study are not randomly distributed as it was for Round 1 interviewing.

Validation of the PHQ-9 and MSPSS for the Current Sample (Aim 1)

As reported in the Method Chapter, while both the PHQ-9 and MSPSS have been validated for use in Uganda in prior studies (Akena, Joska, Obuku, & Stein, 2013; Nakku et al., 2016; Nakigudde, Musisi, Ehnvall, Airaksinen & Agren, 2009), the current sample was notably different from those of these earlier studies with regard to setting, ethnicity, resources and historical context. It was therefore important to evaluate these measures' validity and psychometric properties for the current study. Furthermore, in light of the characteristic of high illiteracy rates among women in Northern Uganda and cognitive impairment being a distinctive feature of depression among women in rural Uganda (Uganda Bureau of Statistics, 2017; Fischer, Ramaswamy, Fischer-Flores & Mugisha, 2018), local mental health professionals recommended modifications to both instruments, which included (1) reducing the time period by the PHQ-9 from 2 weeks to1 week to limit inaccurate recall of symptom frequency; (2) improving the acceptability of the PHQ-9 response options by making the language used more concrete (e.g., changing response option "Not at all" to"0 days," "several days" to "1 to 3 days,"

etc.); and (3) collapsing the 7-point likert scale of the original MSPSS instrument into a 2-tiered,

dichotomized response option model. These modifications to the PHQ-9 and MSPSS also

warranted assessing their validity for the current sample.

The Aim 1 hypotheses that both the PHQ-9 and the MSPSS would maintain their original

factor structures for this sample were confirmed. Reliability analyses for the PHQ-9 indicated the

scale achieved excellent internal consistency in this sample, and all extraction methods from both

the exploratory and confirmatory factor analyses indicated a unidimensional factor structure.

This finding is consistent with studies evaluating the psychometric properties of the Luganda

version of the PHQ-9 as well as other validation studies from the East African region (Akena,

Joska, Obuku, & Stein, 2013; Nakku et al., 2016; Gelaye et al., 2013; Omoro, Fann, Weymuller,

Macharia & Yueh, 2006). The higher Cronbach's alpha value found in this study compared to

other studies in this region may be an indication that the modifications made to this scale

increased its reliability.

The current literature features a handful of studies evaluating the psychometric properties

of the MSPSS in SSA, the findings for which are much less consistent compared to those

assessing the validity of the PHQ-9. Similar to our findings, Nakigudde and colleagues (2009)

found the MSPSS had acceptable internal consistency and maintained its original factor structure

in their Ugandan sample; Dambi and colleagues (Dambi, Tapera, Chiwaridzo, Tadyanemhandu,

& Nhunzvi, 2017), however, found that a two-factor structure merging the family and significant

other subscales was a better fit for their Zimbabwean sample. Findings on the Hausa version of

the scale in a Nigerian sample follow a similar pattern, where a two-factor structure of friends and family (family and significant other subscales) is deemed acceptable over the original three-factor model (Mohammad, Al Sadat, Loh, & Chinna, 2015). This may be attributable to conclusions drawn in the literature and summarized by Dambi and others, which state that "family" and "special persons" (i.e., intimate partners) are often seen as conceptually indistinguishable in SSA cultures (Dambi, Tapera, Chiwaridzo, Tadyanemhandu, & Nhunzvi, 2017).

Interestingly, Aloba, Opakunle, and Ogunrinu (2019) find that the original factor structure best fits their Nigerian sample of adolescents from the Southwestern region. This differential finding may be related to characteristics of this sample, namely their youth. Given that adolescents are in a different life stage where marriage is often uncommon, it is likely that discrimination between significant others and family members and the role they play in adolescents' lives is more apparent.

The original factor structure of the MSPSS was found acceptable in the Malawian sample studied by Stewart, Umar, Tomenson & Creed (2014) as well; however, goodness-of-fit differed by language. Stewart and colleagues found that the MSPSS original factor structure was more appropriate for Chichewa speakers than for Chiyao speakers. It should also be noted that a principal components analysis rather than the recommended exploratory factor analysis was run in this study to determine the number of extracted factors. This conflicts with the statistical approach most readily recommended by the literature (Thompson & Daniel, 1996; Costello & Osborne, 2005; Izquierdo, Diaz, & Garcia, 2014).

Differences in Rates of Maternal Behaviors Promoting Child Health in Probably Depressed and Nondepressed Mothers (Aim 2)

Aim 2 of the current study was to critically assess differences between probably depressed and nondepressed mothers in their endorsement of child health promoting behaviors and in child health outcomes. The behavior and health domains explored included the following: (1) integrated management of childhood illness; (2) infant and young child feeding practices; (3) water, sanitation and hygiene behaviors; (4) child illness prevention practices; and (5) child health outcomes. While just over half of the hypothesized behaviors were found to hold significant relationships with probable depression, some of these relationships were associated in the opposite direction than was expected. As a result, some hypotheses were only partially confirmed.

Integrated management of childhood illness. The aim 2a hypothesis stating that seeking advice or treatment for child illness within 24 hours and knowing at least three danger signs of childhood illness would be negatively associated with probable depression was only partially confirmed. While nondepressed mothers were, as expected, more likely than their probably depressed counterparts to seek advice or treatment for their sick child within 24 hours (as recommended by the World Health Organization), probably depressed mothers demonstrated a higher average number of known danger signs of child illness, contrary to our prediction.

This finding begins to address a gap in the literature examining the relationships between maternal depression and IMCI behaviors. To our knowledge, ours is the first study to examine the association between depression and knowledge of danger signs of childhood illness. Probably depressed mothers' greater knowledge of danger signs may be a reflection of the maternal preoccupation common in maternal mental illness, which has been shown to reduce parental responsiveness (Stein, Lehtonen, Harvey, Nicol-Harper, & Craske, 2009). Interestingly, the probably depressed women in our study were able to identify on average more danger signs of neonatal and childhood illness than general population participants in a number of studies carried out in East African samples, where average knowledge settled around one to two danger signs (Sandberg, Petterson, Asp, Kabakyenga & Agardh, 2014; Berhane, Yimam, Jibat & Zewdu, 2018; Alemu-Guta, Sema, Amsalu, & Sintayehu, 2020; Nigatu, Worku, & Dadi, 2015; Kibaru & Otara, 2016).

Importantly, however, the current study indicates that the presence of depression complicates the assumption that greater knowledge of danger signs will naturally lead to quicker or more effective treatment-seeking behavior. For mothers with probable depression, despite knowing more danger signs they were less likely to seek care for their child within 24 hours. This finding offers direction for further studies seeking to clarify the mechanism that delays treatment-seeking for sick children by depressed mothers.

It is important to emphasize the association both poor knowledge of danger signs and delayed care-seeking have with neonatal death. Sandberg and colleagues found that in Uganda, poor knowledge was associated with delayed care-seeking for the sick child, which accounts for about half of all neonatal death in eastern Uganda (Sandberg, Petterson, Asp, Kabakyenga & Agardh, 2014). The researchers found that half of their study sample reported delayed recognition of the child's health concern or a delay in the decision to seek care for their child. These findings emphasize the importance of pinpointing the missing link in Ugandan mothers' help-seeking for their sick children. The current study's findings on the associations among maternal depression, knowledge, and treatment-seeking help to initiate that search. Despite probably depressed mothers' demonstration of greater knowledge of danger signs of childhood illness, their seeking of care for their sick child remains delayed compared to their nondepressed counterparts. This may be a reflection of the limits to functioning maternal depression can impose on a mother. Fatigue, poor attention and concentration, sluggishness are all common symptoms of postpartum depression that can interfere with a mother's ability to act on important knowledge about the integrated management of childhood illness.

It is also important to note this study's finding of a significant association between probable depression and the rate of childhood illness. These findings are corroborated by research on maternal depression and rates of child diarrhea in Nigeria. Adewuya and others (Adewuya, Ola, Aloba, Mapayi, & Okeniyi, 2008) found that by 9 months postpartum, the children of depressed mothers had on average experienced a significantly greater number of diarrheal episodes than the children of their nondepressed counterparts. In rural Pakistan as well, the children of depressed mothers were more than twice as likely to have had at least five diarrheal episodes in 1 year compared to the children of nondepressed women (Rahman, Bunn, Lovel & Creed, 2007).

A number of studies have converged on the finding that postpartum depression distinctly bears a significant association with increased risk for diarrheal episodes (Adewuya, Aloba, Mapayi, & Okeniyi, 2008; Okronipa et al., 2012; Gausia, Ali & Ryder, 2010; Ndokera & MacArthur, 2011; Weobong et al., 2015). Such an association is not evident for ante- or perinatal depression (Waqas et al., 2015), indicating the important role treating postpartum depression in particular plays in improving child health. As numerous studies have emphasized, diarrhea among infants can lead to severe malnourishment and far too often, neonatal death if left untreated (Kosek, Bern & Guerrant, 2003; Bryce, Boschi-Pinto, Shibuya, Black & WHO Child Health Epidemiology Reference Group, 2005; Mukuku et al., 2019; Schlaudecker, Steinhoff, & Moore, 2011). This presents a strong case for addressing the factors that interfere with mothers' seeking treatment for their children. The urgency is that much greater for mothers who are depressed.

Infant and young child feeding practices. Our second hypothesis for Aim 2 of this study was not confirmed; within this sample, no significant differences were found between probably depressed and nondepressed mothers in reported rates of breastfeeding for children younger than six months and reported rates of six to 23 month old children meeting minimum dietary diversity criteria. Because no nondepressed women in this sample endorsed providing their child more fluids than usual during illness, the difference between groups for this practice could not be analyzed. While a difference was found between groups for whether a child was fed the same amount or more food than usual during illness, the association fell in the opposite direction of our expectation: depressed women reported providing their child the same amount or more food than usual to their sick child at higher rates than their nondepressed counterparts.

Of all IYCF practices, breastfeeding indicators are certainly the most researched in the context of PPD. Though most studies exploring this topic identify PPD as a predictor of early breastfeeding cessation, reduced breastfeeding frequency or failure to initiate breastfeeding, it is important to note that the majority of this research was performed in HIC settings (Dennis &

McQueen, 2007; McLearn, Minkovitz, Strobino, Marks, & Hou, 2006; Henderson, Evans,

Straton, Priest, & Hagan, 2003; Bogen, Hanusa, Moses-Kolko & Wisner, 2010).

In low-income communities, findings are far less uniform. Consistent with the current

study's findings, a number of researchers have found no significant relationship between PPD

and breastfeeding variables (McKee, Zayas, & Jankowski, 2004; Farias-Antunez, Santos,

Matijasevich, & de Barros, 2020; Chung, McCollum, Elo, Lee, & Culhane, 2004).

Perhaps most importantly, the current study's finding of an insignificant association

between PPD and exclusive breastfeeding is consistent with the systematic review and meta-

analysis conducted by Handiso et al. (2020), which evaluated the relationship between these

variables of interest in SSA countries, including 26 studies from nine countries across Eastern,

Western and Southern Africa. Interestingly, despite pooled prevalence rates of 18.6%, 20.2% and

18.5%, respectively, for these subregions, which exceeded the WHO report for the prevalence of

PPD in 2018, the findings in these SSA countries are in conflict with much of the evidence found

to support this association in other areas of the world. The trend of insignificant findings in

resource-poor communities when examining the association between PPD and breastfeeding

behaviors may be an indication that the effects of depressive symptoms are subsumed under the

more generalized burden of poverty. Women in SSA regions like those in our sample may

prioritize components of effective child care and health promotion differently from those in more

privileged communities. For these women, breastfeeding may be considered a high-expenditure,

low-reward activity considering the time and energy required to maintain this behavior that could

otherwise be spent working in their garden or tending to the household, activities that may feel

beneficial to the greater family unit. This prospect is supported by studies that show the likelihood of exclusive breastfeeding increases as income increases (McCarter-Spaulding &.

Horowitz, 2007; Moran et al., 2015), and early introduction of complementary foods is

associated with low socioeconomic status (Tatone-Tokuda, Dubois & Girard, 2009; Baydar,

McCann, Willliams, & Vesper, 1997; Heinig et al., 2006).

Outside of breastfeeding as well, research examining the relationships between PPD and

IYCF paints a complex, and at times, conflictual picture. In one of the few papers observing

mothers' feeding practices for their ill children, Singer et al. (1996) found that mothers

presenting with depressive or anxiety symptoms who had a child with very low birth weight and

bronchopulmonary dysplasia decreased their verbal prompting of their infants to feed after the

child demonstrated non-feeding behavior. This may be an indication of mothers with mental

health symptoms being less engaged in the practices of IYCF compared to their asymptomatic

counterparts. This stands in conflict with our study's finding that depressed women report

feeding their sick child the same or more than the usual amount of food at higher rates than

nondepressed women.

A study examining the role of maternal worries in the relationship between disordered

child feeding and mother-child feeding interactions may offer some explanation for this finding.

Gueron-Sela, Aztaba-Poria, Meiri, and Yerushalmi (2011) found that maternal worries about

child underweight both mediated and moderated this relationship; the researchers found that

mothers of children with feeding disorders were prone to greater intrusiveness and less

structuring during feeding interactions. Their findings lend support to the report from Chatoor

Hirsch, and Persinger (1997) that mothers who are vulnerable to worry experience increased

anxiety when their child refuses to eat, and as a result they may engage in forceful feeding. This maternal worry may contribute to the symptom profile of maternal depression in this current

sample, where depressed mothers of sick children may have increased the child's consumption

by virtue of her worry and forceful feeding.

Two other important considerations when contextualizing this peculiar finding are both

the quality and the timing of these feedings of sick children and how they may ultimately

reinforce child illness. Madlala and Kassier (2018) importantly highlight the elevated risk of

infant exposure to infectious disease through the premature introduction of solid foods. This risk

is of particular concern for the children of depressed women, as Anato, Baye, Tafese and

Stoecker (2020) report the finding from their Ethopian sample that women with PPD

demonstrate a greater likelihood of introducing complementary foods earlier than is

recommended when compared to their nondepressed counterparts. These researchers additionally

note that depression could impair mothers' abilities to provide nutritious meals for their children.

This is consistent with our own finding that not having depression was positively associated with

the number of nutrient-dense and fortified complementary foods fed to one's child in the

previous 24-hour period. In other words, while our findings may indicate that depressed women

are reporting feeding their sick child more frequently than their nondepressed counterparts,

attention must be paid to the quality and timing of these feedings. This practice may be

increasing the child's vulnerability to illness through early introduction of complementary

feeding and failing to provide the child with the necessary nutrients to fight infection. Further

qualitative research is needed to understand differences in beliefs, practices, motivation and

obstacles faced by depressed and nondepressed women in implementing practices consistent

with IYCF guidelines.

Water, sanitation and hygiene behaviors. The current study's results partially confirmed

hypothesis 2c, which stated the availability of a soap-and-water hand-washing station in the

home, use of a safe disposal method for child fecal matter and use of an adequate treatment

method of household drinking water would be negatively associated with probable depression.

As predicted, women with probable depression reported use of a safe disposal method for child

feces at lower rates than nondepressed women.

Unexpectedly, however, the relationships of probable depression with both availability of a

handwashing station in the home and use of an adequate water treatment method were both

significant and positive, such that probably depressed women endorsed both of these health-

promoting behaviors at higher rates.

To our knowledge, this is the first study to investigate and identify a positive relationship

between poor sanitation and hygiene practices and postpartum depression, lending support to the

framework Stewart (2007) proposed to clarify the mechanisms underlying the relationship

between maternal depression and poor infant growth. As Stewart summarily notes in his review,

depressed mothers are consistently found to provide poorer-quality care across a number of

domains, including care-seeking practices, feeding, cognitive stimulation and attachment

(Stewart, 2007). Our finding adds to the array of research highlighting areas in which depressed

mothers are in need of support to provide comprehensive care for their children, and it indicates

that further research is warranted to clarify the extent to which poor hygienic practices are

contributing to the more severely negative outcomes for these children.

As George and associates (2016) indicate through the findings of their prospective

cohort study of children in a rural Bangladeshi community, households utilizing unsafe disposal methods for child fecal matter show significantly higher environmental enteropathy scores and have children who demonstrate reduced growth rates with regard to weight-for-age and weight-for-height and demonstrate greater odds of wasting. Their findings are consistent with those of Brown and colleagues (2013) that children in low-income countries are the most vulnerable to enteric infection.

As the United Nations describes in its rationale for its sixth sustainable development goal of access to clean water and sanitation for all people, close to 1.8 billion people worldwide drink from a fecally contaminated water source, and 2.4 billion do not have access to basic sanitation services (Bain et al., 2014; Berendes, Sumner, & Brown, 2017). The unfortunate majority of these populations are living in African countries, with an estimated 577 million people in this region living without appropriate management of fecal sludge (Berendes, Sumner, & Brown, 2017).

Wang et al. (2017), in their investigation of exposure of children under 5 to fecal contamination in Ghana, indicate that children 1 to 2 years of age may be particularly vulnerable to enteric infection. Children 0 to 1 year old, who are more likely to be exclusively breastfed, benefit from some protection against exposure via food pathways, which the authors found to be the primary means of transmission for these pathogens. Children 2 to 5 years, while the age group facing the greatest likelihood of exposure, often have greater immunity as a result of prior infection. They therefore tend to require exposure at greater doses to suffer negative health outcomes compared to younger children. Children 1 to 2 years of age are in the unique position of having been introduced to complementary feeding, increased mobility, which increases their floor contact compared to other age groups, and all while toting a very fragile immune system.

Findings from Knee and others (2018) lend support to this interpretation, showing that diarrheal disease was highest among children 12 -23 months within their sample of under-five Mozambican children. Rates were also higher among boys compared to girls.

Maternal depression's counterintuitive relationships with availability of a handwashing statement and use of an adequate water treatment method is easily explained by an inescapable factor within the methodology of the study: access to water. Because full baseline interviews for probably depressed and nondepressed were administered at different times, and in different seasons, the differences in conditions and access to resources across these time points must be considered. As Check (2015) and others indicate, the dry season in SSA is known to severely limit a household's income, food security, and access to water (Onyiriuka, 2006, Friis et al., 2004). With handwashing and drinking water treatment being two water-based activities, a likely explanation for the differences we found between groups in these behaviors was that women will practice these behaviors at higher rates during the rainy season, regardless of depression status, when water is a more plentiful resource.

The current study's findings add texture to the extant literature. The collection of data at different time points for probably depressed and nondepressed women compromises our ability to make sound interpretations about the relationship between maternal depression and water-based health practices; however, our findings begin to expose the underpinnings of the consistent link found between maternal depression and negative child health outcomes like diarrheal illness by identifying unsafe disposal of child feces as an underlying mechanism at play in this relationship.

Child illness prevention behaviors. Due to the sparse data bias explained in the results chapter for child illness prevention behaviors, Hypothesis 2d for this study was unable to be tested. More data is needed to determine whether probable depression is significantly associated with use of an insecticide-treated net for children under 2 years of age. Of note, however, probable depression was determined to not be significantly related to whether a mother monitored her child's growth.

The only study found to examine how maternal depression relates to use of an insecticide treated net found that Ghanaian women with antenatal depression were less likely to use this item during pregnancy (Weobong et al., 2014). No significant difference was found between women with and without antenatal depression regarding their likelihood of putting their infant under a treated net, however. Further research on the association of maternal depression with both mother and child's use of an insecticide-treated net is crucial, as placental malaria has been shown to result in significant obstetric complications that threaten the lives of newborns, including stillbirth, preterm birth, low birth weight, and small size for gestational age (Zakama, Ozarslan & Gaw, 2020). Placental malaria also increases the child's susceptibility to the disease (Harrington et al., 2017), which can result in fatal consequences for the children in the age group captured by the current study. As the WHO World Malaria Report indicates, the majority of deaths from malaria occur among children under 5 (WHO, 2019).

Child health outcomes. Contributing to the wide body of literature linking maternal depression to poorer child health outcomes, the results of the current study confirmed hypothesis 2e, predicting a negative association would be identified between probable depression and child underweight. No association was found in support of hypothesis 2f, however, anticipating an association in the same direction between probable depression and child stunting.

Of the children for whom reliable anthropometric measurements were taken in this study, 29.8% met the WHO criteria for stunting (defined as height-for-age z-score greater than two standard deviations below the mean), and 27.5% for underweight (defined as weight-for-age z-score greater than two standard deviations below the mean). While the stunting rate for this sample is in line with the national prevalence of 29%, based on data from the 2016 Uganda Demographic and Health Survey, the current study's rate for child underweight found in this study far exceeded the 11% estimate national prevalence (Uganda Bureau of Statistics, 2017). This difference may be attributable to the current study's sampling from a more rural and poverty-stricken portion of the Ugandan population, where child malnutrition may be more common. It may also be related to the over-representation of depressed mothers in this sample.

The significant relationship between probable depression and one child health outcome but not the other is puzzling, though not outstanding from the current literature from the SSA region, where the association of maternal depression to child health outcomes like underweight and stunting is less consistent than in the South and Southeast Asian contexts (Parsons, Young, Rochat, Kringelbach, & Stein, 2012). In South Africa, for example, Christodoulou and colleagues (2020) identify no associations between perinatal maternal depression and negative child growth outcomes at birth or at 2 years, findings which corroborate the results of one of the earliest studies on this topic within the SSA context, run by Cooper and associates (1999). Avan and colleagues (2010), however, yield disparate findings in their own longitudinal birth cohort study. They identified the children of depressed mothers to be at about a 60% greater risk for stunting at 2 years of age compared to those of nondepressed mothers. The reason for these divergent results is difficult to determine.

Conflicting results are found in Northern Ghana as well. Wemakor and Iddrisu (2018) failed to find evidence to support a significant association between maternal depression and stunting; interestingly, the same first author found depressed mothers in the same region to be nearly three times as likely to have a stunted child in a paper published 2 years earlier (Wemakor & Mensah, 2016). The opposing findings may be attributable to differences between studies in child age groups. While maternal depression did not significantly relate to stunting among children 6 to 23 months of age, the association appeared to have been made evident within children 0 to 59 months. A similar pattern may be at work within the population from which the current study's sample was taken, where the association between these constructs does not become apparent until after the child's first 2 years of life.

To our knowledge, only two studies examine the relationship between maternal mental health and child health outcomes in Uganda. Counterintuitively, Ickes, Wu, Mandel and Roberts (2018) find that as a mother's psychological satisfaction increases, her likelihood of having a child who is stunted also increases. Ashaba and associates (2015), however, yield findings in line with the expected direction of this relationship. They found maternal depression was positively associated with malnutrition. A shortcoming of this study, however, is that stunting and underweight are not examined separately but are instead aggregated into a single malnutrition indicator.

As we seek to clarify the relationship between maternal mental health and child malnutrition within the SSA context, the current study's findings, which add to the complexity of the SSA literature, appear to indicate the need to split from the tradition in global mental health research of superimposing maternal and child health observations made within South and Southeast Asian cultures onto African populations. Though as of 2019, stunting rates in these regions are comparable both in percentage and number of children under 5 affected, with about 33-34% of children in each region experiencing reduced linear growth, a significant downward trend in rates within South Asian populations have occurred since 1990, while rates in Africa have increased (De Onis & Branca, 2016; Vaivada et al., 2020). These trends speak to the urgency of understanding the unique and inconsistent link between malnutrition and maternal depression as it appears in SSA.

Moderating Role of Perceived Social Support (Aim 3)

To our surprise, perceived social support was found to be of little consequence as a moderator in the relationships between postpartum depression and child health promoting behaviors and outcomes. Only hypothesis 3a was found to be partially confirmed through the significant interaction found between probable depression and perceived social support for availability of a soap-and-water handwashing station in the home. Depressed participants with low perceived social support had lower odds of having a handwashing station in the home while probably depressed participants with high perceived social support had higher odds of having this resource. This finding is partially explained by the issue of water-availability, as previously discussed.

While the current study did not find a significant interaction between depression and social support for any of the IYCF indicators, findings from Ickes and colleagues on the relationships social support and maternal psychological health hold with these health promoting behaviors can be of aid in interpreting our understanding of the association of social support with health promoting behaviors more broadly (Ickes, Wu, Mandel and Roberts, 2018). Having found that social support was positively associated with each of the IYCF indicators they assessed, these researchers posited that greater social support may facilitate knowledge and skill-sharing within a mother's network, thereby increasing her use of health-promoting practices. This dynamic may be at play within the current sample as well, such that women with access to social support may activate their network to a greater extent than when not depressed, which increases the aforementioned exchange of knowledge and resources.

The moderating effect of social support in this relationship may also pertain to the amount of instrumental support a mother receives, which may have been partially captured by MSPSS items (i.e., Item 3: My family really tries to help me; Item 6: My friends really try to help me; Item 7: I can count on my friends when things go wrong). As indicated by Hadley and colleagues (2007) and Tsai et al. (2011) , women residing in resource-poor and food-insecure settings similar to the current study may find that of the four types of social support, which include emotional, informational, companionship and instrumental, the latter has the most meaningful impact on their lives (Cohen, Underwood & Gottlieb, 2000). Importantly, mothers' perceived instrumental support has been found to maintain a positive association with their children's overall health above and beyond the effects of a mother's economic security and general wellbeing, when examining this relationship in a sample with an over-representation of minority and economically disadvantaged families (Turney, 2013).

Moderating Role of Women's Empowerment Indicators (Aim 4)

Aim 4 of the current study sought to investigate the impact of mothers' perceived empowerment (as measured by indicators of household decision-making, attitudes toward intimate partner violence, and contraception use) on child health promoting behaviors and child health outcomes. Attitudes toward intimate partner violence and contraception use were each found to meaningfully moderate the relationships probable depression had with at least two child health promoting behaviors, therefore partially confirming Hypothesis 4a, while household decision-making was a moderator for none. For child underweight and stunting, none of these indicators moderated its relationship with probable depression. The current study therefore failed to confirm Hypotheses 4b and 4c. These findings are contextualized in the current literature below.

Household decision-making. Our insignificant findings for the moderating role of household decision-making is consistent with the current literature, providing evidence to suggest that household decision-making is not an appropriate indicator for women's empowerment in the SSA context (Upadhyay and Karasek, 2012; Schatz and Williams, 2012). As Upadhyay and Karasek suggest in their study of women's empowerment and ideal family size in four SSA countries, attitudes toward intimate partner violence may provide a more accurate picture of women's empowerment in the SSA context compared to household decision-making, which has been found to perform well in South and Southeast Asia but appears to be of scant significance in SSA countries (Upadhyay and Karasek, 2012).

Attitudes toward intimate partner violence. Attitudes toward intimate partner violence was found to meaningfully interact with probable depression only among women reporting lower acceptance of IPV, such that depressed women with low acceptance of IPV were more likely to take longer to seek care for their sick child but also more likely to have a handwashing station in the household compared to their nondepressed counterparts. This finding may be a consequence of greater conflict within the intimate relationships of partnered women with less accepting attitudes toward IPV. Interestingly, Ahinkorah, Dickson and Seidu (2018) consolidate findings from multiple studies of IPV in SSA, which report that women who are more empowered are more likely to suffer from IPV. This is possibly due to these women's refusal to be subordinate to their husbands, which may lead to increased marital conflict. It may also be the case in our findings that due to conflict with their partners, whose financial contributions are often necessary to be able to afford health care for a sick child, depressed women with low IPV acceptance are unable to access treatment for their sick child as quickly as healthy comparisons.

Contraception Use. Our finding that among women who deny using contraception, depressed women are more likely to have a handwashing station is more difficult to understand, however, particularly given that women who endorse contraception use were more likely to have a handwashing facility in their household regardless of depression status. The same interaction trend was found for the amount of food offered to a sick child. For both outcomes the main effect of contraception use may be at play, where a woman who is empowered (i.e., endorsing contraception use) is more likely to have a handwashing station in her home and feed her child the same or more food than usual regardless of her depression status. While a woman who is not depressed and disempowered is least likely to report engaging in these health promoting practices, a disempowered woman who is also depressed may be activating her social support system to participate more intensively in childcare activities. As Alem, Jacobsson and Hanlon (2008) point out, in traditional SSA societies, family and community members play a pivotal role in provision of care for people struggling with mental illness, noting that social support in this region tends to be greater than in the West. If families view their mentally ill members as their responsibility, it is likely that members are stepping in to take care of the day-to-day needs of these depressed women, including caring for their children.

Limitations

There are several limitations to the current study and the parent study from which the data analyzed was taken, including issues of methodological design and operationalization of our variables of interest. These limitations are presented below.

Time Differences in Data Collection

The primary factor complicating the interpretation of maternal depression's association with child health-promoting behaviors is the time difference in the collection of data for the probably depressed and nondepressed groups. Because nondepressed women participated in the full baseline interview up to 2 months after data were collected for probably depressed mothers, issues such as seasonality, water availability, and differences in child age complicated the picture of maternal behavior in the presence or absence of depressive symptoms. Particularly in Uganda,

167

where the rainy and dry seasons have profound impacts on the day-to-day lives of women and resource-availability, it is crucial to consider potential effects of one's environment on a mother's mental health, her child's health, and her household.

Differences in child age at the time of interview may also have influenced mothers' experiences with depressive symptoms and the extent to which mothers endorsed the practices within each behavioral domain. For example, a mother's beliefs related to infant feeding practices for a six-month old may differ considerably from those held for an 8-month old. The extent of a mother's involvement in child feeding, the perceived impact of the child's dependence, and cultural expectations related to family member participation in caretaking at these ages may contribute to differences in maternal workload or perceived psychological burden. It is therefore of the utmost importance for concurrent data collection to take place when comparing depressed and nondepressed women and for seasonal differences to be accounted for when comparing these groups.

Unbalanced Design

An additional complication in the analysis of these data was utilization of an unbalanced design. Given the nearly four-fold over-representation of probably depressed women in the current sample, drawing comparisons between groups for both demographic characteristics and health-promoting behaviors was made difficult. With such a limited sample of nondepressed women, making definitive conclusions about possible risk and protective factors for depression among mothers in this area was infeasible. While use of a balanced design is most recommended, an alternative solution is use of a weighting technique to achieve balanced sampling and meet assumptions of generalizability.

Cross-Sectional Design

An additional limitation of the current-study was analysis of cross-sectional data, which does not allow for determination of causality within relationships between variables. As a result, while it is possible that a mother's depressive symptoms are interfering with her ability to care for her child, which increases the child's likelihood of illness, the causality of this relationship may move in the opposite direction as well, where a child's increased likelihood of illness causes depressive symptoms in his mother. Having set a solid foundation from which future studies can build, it will be important for additional research examining the significant relationships found in the current study to adopt a longitudinal design.

Self-Report

The current study's use of a self-report surveying procedure is an additional limitation to be considered. While self-report is both a convenient and frequently utilized approach in global mental health research, this method inevitably makes a study vulnerable to recall and social desirability biases, particularly within study contexts such as this one, where participation often is associated with the promise of resources in the form of compensation or connection with well-resourced humanitarian organizations. In the absence of direct observations of mothers' interactions with and care for their child, it is difficult to confirm the veracity of their reports. These biases may also have been at play in mothers' reports of their experiences with depressive symptoms. It is therefore advised that future studies consider collecting data in part by means of direct observation and/or key informants.

Convenience Sampling for Round 2 Interviewing

As aforementioned in the methods chapter, a convenience sampling method was employed for Round 2 interviewing of nondepressed mothers, based on the availability of participants and their proximity to the enumerators' locations. Because our catchment area covered a large amount of land with rough terrain, transportation options were limited. As a result, second round interviewing was confined to those sub-counties more easily reached by independent enumerators. While use of this method was necessary to obtain full baseline data on nondepressed participants, it has posed limitations to the generalizability of our findings, and it creates some difficulty in making demographic comparisons of nondepressed and depressed participants, the latter group having been recruited using a cluster random sampling method.

Operationalization

The following section discusses limitations related to the operationalization of our independent variables of interest, probable depression, perceived social support, and women's empowerment indicators.

Maternal Depression. Maternal depression was operationalized by a score of 10 or greater on the PHQ-9, a commonly used and well-validated screener for major depression (Kroenke, Spitzer & Willians, 2001; Akena, Joska, Obuku, & Stein, 2013; Nakku et al., 2016). Informed by the clinical insights of local mental health professionals with whom we collaborated in Uganda, we

170

decided to modify the PHQ-9 to report frequency of depressive symptoms over the last week rather than 2 weeks. Our collaborators suggested this was an important adjustment to make to improve the accuracy of participant recall of symptoms; however, this eliminated the possibility of our ability to assess for the occurrence of major depression as defined by the American Psychiatric Association (2013). As a result, throughout this text, we referred to a score of 10 or greater as probable depression.

Additionally, data were not available in the current study confirming the onset of depressive symptoms. The onset specifier for depression with peripartum onset delineated in the American Psychiatric Association's Diagnostic and Statistical Manual of Mental Disorders, fifth edition is within 4 weeks postpartum (2013). Probable maternal depression is defined for this study as within the first 2 years postpartum. This modification as well as the adjusted time frame covered by the PHQ-9 for this study in the absence of comparison to a gold standard may limit the comparability of our findings to other studies of maternal depression.

Another important consideration regarding the operationalization of the condition examined in the current study is the potential self-limiting nature of the term "maternal depression." On one hand, the symptoms screened for using the PHQ-9 may be capturing a condition within maternal mental health with a more expansive definition than depression is able to provide; on the other, by narrowing our focus to maternal depression exclusively, we may have failed to capture meaningful symptoms of maternal psychological distress that extend beyond the scope of depression but still contribute to the extent of a mother's engagement in child health-promoting behaviors. In future studies, it will be important to cast a wider net in terms of symptomatology, emphasizing other important categories of common perinatal mental health disorders (CPMDs), particularly anxiety.

Finally, the inconsistent moderating effects of perceived social support and women's empowerment indicators may be highlighting subtypes of depression. As described in Nolen-Hoeksema's (1991) Response Styles Theory, there may have been a group of probably depressed participants who responded to their depressed mood with adaptive reflection rather than maladaptive brooding. Use of this coping style may have allowed this group of mothers to more readily engage in the health-promoting behaviors this study investigated.

Perceived Social Support. Perceived social support was measured using the MSPSS, previously validated for use among postpartum mothers in Uganda, but with some modification (Nakigudde, Musisi, Ehnvall, Airaksinen & Agren, 2009). In our study as well, modifications to the Likert scale response options were found acceptable to this sample. However, the collapsing of the measure's original 7-point likert scale into a 2-tiered, dichotomized response option model for the current study removed the neutral response option. This change may have forced participants to agree or disagree with items on which they held no opinion, which may have resulted in biased data.

Implications and Future Directions

Despite the above-listed limitations, implications of the current study's findings and directions for further study are substantial. Findings from the current study contribute to the evidence of a strong relationship existing between maternal depression and adverse child health outcomes. Being only the third study to have examined this relationship in Uganda, our findings are impactful in helping us to understand the contours of this relationship when tailored uniquely to the Ugandan context. While much of the research on child malnutrition has emphasized child stunting, our findings highlight the threat maternal depression may pose to child survival by means of child underweight, to which about 53% of child deaths per year can be attributed (Harpham, Huttly, De Silva, & Abramsky, 2005; Black, Morris, & Bryce, 2003). For this reason, and informed by our finding of probable depression being associated with both having a sick child and feeding a sick child the same amount or more food than usual, we recommend that future studies involve detailed inquiry of both the quality and quantity of food being offered to children. It is also advised that qualitative data be gathered to better understand what beliefs and considerations may inform mothers' IYCF practices.

Furthermore, our study identified an important and counterintuitive disparity regarding IMCI behaviors: despite depressed mothers having demonstrated greater knowledge of danger signs of childhood illness, they were slower to seek out treatment for their sick children. Being the first study to examine the relationship between maternal depression and danger sign knowledge, this finding makes evident that education is not the missing link in effective management of childhood illness for depressed mothers. To improve child health promoting behaviors in this domain, our results indicate that treatment of maternal depression is crucial.

Similarly, no other study has examined how maternal depression relates to WASH behaviors within SSA in such a detailed manner. Our finding that depressed women report lower rates of utilizing safe child feces disposal methods, possibly due to safe methods requiring more planning and effort, could meaningfully contribute to community-based interventions targeting both maternal depression and sanitation and hygiene promotion interventions in Uganda. Given this difference between depressed and nondepressed mothers, it would be important to engage depressed mothers in recruiting support from loved ones to help with consistent use of these hygienic practices.

Future studies investigating the relationship between maternal depression and WASH behaviors in Uganda should also be careful to consider seasonality as a confounding variable. In the current study, seasonality was likely a major explanatory variable for the differences we saw between groups for water treatment and handwashing practices. In fact, seasonality may make important contributions to maternal mood itself. In rural Ghana, delivering a child during the dry season was identified as a risk factor for PPD over and above the effects of AND, adverse birth outcomes and obstetric complications (Weobong et al., 2015). The authors cite increased risk of child illness and child care difficulties unique to this season as possible explanations for the risk this time of year poses to mothers.

In Uganda as well, the dry season presents significant threats to an already poverty-stricken community. In a qualitative study on the effects of seasonality on perinatal health, Ugandan women reported food scarcity and difficult working conditions due to heat as factors impacting their health during the dry season, while the rainy season presents its own challenges, including overexertion from physical labor. Regarding the dry season's food insecurity, one participant stated, "We don't have those foods, that's why we produce smaller babies," and "that's the reason why our babies die in our stomach, because we don't have food" (MacVicar et al.,

2017). Just as we found, an association between maternal depression and poor child health outcomes has consistently been identified in cross-sectional studies in LMIC settings (Ndokera & MacArthur, 2011; Anato, Baye, Tafese & Stoecker, 2020; Wemakor & Mensah, 2016); however, the direction of this relationship cannot be identified. Considering the profound adverse child health outcomes that Ugandan women appear to associate with the dry season, it is plausible that a woman who delivers during this season would experience depressive symptoms about or in anticipation of child health concerns.

Perceived social support is another area warranting further research based on our findings. While the current study found social support as measured by the MSPSS to interact with depression when availability of a handwashing facility is the outcome variable, such that high levels of social support increased depressed women's likelihood of endorsing this behavior, no other significant findings were yielded beyond that. As discussed in the study limitations, the MSPSS only captures one dimension of social support, and perhaps not the type most meaningful to women in SSA cultures. In future studies it would be important to examine the mediating and moderating roles of social support to the relationship between maternal depression and health promoting behaviors, measuring practical and instrumental social support rather than emotional. An additional important component of social support would be collecting qualitative data to understand the extent of involvement of a depressed woman's social network in child care and both the quality and quantity of social support she receives.

Additional considerations for future studies of maternal depression and social support include investigating potential deleterious effects of social support to a mother's parenting self-efficacy, particularly as an adverse reaction to stress. In accordance with the formative social

support theories posed by Wortman (1984) and others, receiving social support may be

experienced by the depressed mother as an indication that her own efforts are inferior (Brickman,

Rabinowitz, Karuza, Cohn & Kidder, 1982).

Finally, further research is warranted to clarify the interaction of women's empowerment

with maternal depression. As was seen in our study, empowerment may act as a buffer against

some of the deleterious effects of depression on a mother's provision of care for her child.

Interestingly, certain indicators of empowerment may also present as barriers to engagement in

child health-promoting behaviors, similar to the finding in our study that women with lower

acceptance of IPV take longer to seek care for their child and are less likely to have a

handwashing station in the home. There may be other factors at play confounding the

relationships among women's empowerment, maternal depression and maternal behaviors that

would be important to examine. A second possibility is that women's empowerment acts

differently or is operationalized differently in the SSA context. As we strive to achieve the

second, third and fifth Sustainable Development Goals of zero hunger, good health and

wellbeing and gender equality by 2030, developing a more comprehensive understanding of

women's empowerment tailored to the experiences of women in SSA will be crucial.

REFERENCES

Abbo, C., Ekblad, S., Waako, P., Okello, E., Muhwezi, W., & Musisi, S. (2008). Psychological distress and associated factors among the attendees of traditional healing practices in Jinja and Iganga districts, Eastern Uganda: a cross-sectional study. *International Journal of Mental Health Systems, 2*(16). https://doi.org/10.1186/1752-4458-2-16.

Abiodun, O. A. (2006). Postnatal depression in primary care populations in Nigeria. *General hospital psychiatry, 28*(2), 133-136.

Adewuya, A. O., Eegunranti, A. B., & Lawal, A. M. (2005). Prevalence of postnatal depression in Western Nigerian women: a controlled study. *International Journal of Psychiatry in Clinical Practice, 9*(1), 60-64.

Adewuya, A. O., Ola, B. A., Aloba, O. O., Dada, A. O., & Fasoto, O. O. (2007). Prevalence and correlates of depression in late pregnancy among Nigerian women. *Depression and anxiety, 24*(1), 15-21.

Adewuya, A. O., Ola, B. O., Aloba, O. O., Mapayi, B. M., & Okeniyi, J. A. (2008). Impact of postnatal depression on infants' growth in Nigeria. *Journal of affective disorders, 108*(1-2), 191-193.

Adjiwanou, V., & LeGrand, T. (2014). Gender inequality and the use of maternal healthcare services in rural sub-Saharan Africa. *Health & place, 29*, 67-78.

Affonso, D. D., De, A. K., Horowitz, J. A., & Mayberry, L. J. (2000). An international study exploring levels of postpartum depressive symptomatology. *Journal of psychosomatic research, 49*(3), 207-216.

Agoub, M., Moussaoui, D., & Battas, O. (2005). Prevalence of postpartum depression in a Moroccan sample. *Archives of Women's Mental Health, 8*(1), 37-43.

Ahinkorah, B. O., Dickson, K. S., & Seidu, A. A. (2018). Women decision-making capacity and intimate partner violence among women in sub-Saharan Africa. *Archives of Public Health, 76*(1), 5.

Akena, D., Joska, J., Obuku, E. A., & Stein, D. J. (2013). Sensitivity and specificity of clinician administered screening instruments in detecting depression among HIV-positive individuals in Uganda. *AIDS care, 25*(10), 1245-1252.

Alem, A., Jacobsson, L., & Hanlon, C. (2008). Community-based mental health care in Africa: mental health workers' views. *World Psychiatry, 7*(1), 54.

Alemu Guta, A. S., Amsalu, B., & Sintayehu, Y. (2020). Knowledge of Neonatal Danger Signs and Associated Factors Among Mothers of< 6 Months Old Child in Dire Dawa, Ethiopia: A Community Based Cross-Sectional Study. *International Journal of Women's Health, 12*, 539.

Al Hinai, F. I., & Al Hinai, S. S. (2014). Prospective Study on Prevalence and Risk Factors of Postpartum Depression in Al-Dakhliya Governorate in Oman. *Oman Medical Journal, 29*(3), 198–202. http://doi.org/10.5001/omj.2014.49

Alkire, S., Meinzen-Dick, R., Peterman, A., Quisumbing, A., Seymour, G., & Vaz, A. (2013). The women's empowerment in agriculture index. *World Development, 52*, 71-91.

Aloba, O., Opakunle, T., & Ogunrinu, O. (2019). Psychometric characteristics and measurement invariance across genders of the multidimensional scale of perceived social support (MSPSS) among Nigerian adolescents. *Health Psychology Report, 7*(1), 69-80.

Altemus, M., Sarvaiya, N., & Epperson, C. N. (2014). Sex differences in anxiety and depression clinical perspectives. *Frontiers in neuroendocrinology, 35*(3), 320-330.

American Psychiatric Association. (2013). *Diagnostic and statistical manual of mental disorders* (5th ed.). Washington, DC: Publisher.

Anato, A., Baye, K., Tafese, Z., & Stoecker, B. J. (2020). Maternal depression is associated with child undernutrition: A cross-sectional study in Ethiopia. *Maternal & child nutrition, 16*(3), e12934.

Anderson, J. C., & Gerbing, D. W. (1988). Structural equation modeling in practice: A review and recommended two-step approach. *Psychological bulletin, 103*(3), 411.

Applied Mental Health Research Group. Design, implementation, monitoring, and evaluation of cross-cultural HIV-related mental health and psychosocial assistance programs: A user's manual for researchers and program implementers. Baltimore, Maryland: Unpublished manual, Bloomberg School of Public Health, Johns Hopkins University; 2011.

Arifin, S.R.M, Cheyne, H., & Maxwell, M. (2018). Review of the prevalence of postnatal depression across cultures. *AIMS Public Health, 5*(3), 260-295.

Asaolu, I. O., Alaofè, H., Gunn, J. K., Adu, A. K., Monroy, A. J., Ehiri, J. E., ... & Ernst, K. C. (2018). Measuring women's Empowerment in sub-Saharan Africa: exploratory and confirmatory factor analyses of the demographic and health surveys. *Frontiers in psychology, 9*, 994.

178

Ashaba, S., Kaida, A., Coleman, J. N., Burns, B. F., Dunkley, E., O'Neil, K., ... & Matthews, L. T. (2017). Psychosocial challenges facing women living with HIV during the perinatal period in rural Uganda. *PLoS One, 12*(5), e0176256.

Ashaba, S., Rukundo, G.Z., Beinempaka, F., Ntaro, M., & LeBlanc, J.C. (2015). Maternal depression and malnutrition in children in southwest Uganda: a case control study. *BMC Public Health, 15*(1), 1303-1308.

Avan, B., Richter, L. M., Ramchandani, P. G., Norris, S. A., & Stein, A. (2010). Maternal postnatal depression and children's growth and behaviour during the early years of life: exploring the interaction between physical and mental health. *Archives of disease in childhood, 95*(9), 690-695.

Bain, R., Cronk, R., Hossain, R., Bonjour, S., Onda, K., Wright, J., ... & Bartram, J. (2014). Global assessment of exposure to faecal contamination through drinking water based on a systematic review. *Tropical Medicine & International Health, 19*(8), 917-927.)

Bandiera, O., Buehren, N., Burgess, R., Goldstein, M., Gulesci, S., Rasul, I., & Sulaiman, M. (2015). Women's Economic Empowerment in Action: Evidence from a Randomized Control Trial in Africa.

Baranov, V., Bhalotra, S., Biroli, P., & Maselko, J. (2019). Maternal Depression, Women's Empowerment, and Parental Investment: Evidence from a Randomized Control Trial. *American Economic Review*.

Barber, S. L., & Gertler, P. J. (2009). Health workers, quality of care, and child health: Simulating the relationships between increases in health staffing and child length. *Health policy, 91*(2), 148-155.

Basu, A. M. (1992). *Culture, the status of women, and demographic behaviour: illustrated with the case of India*. Clarendon Press.

Baydar, N., McCann, M., Williams, R., & Vesper, E. (1997). WIC infant feeding practices study. Final report. Alexandria, VA: USDA, Food and Nutrition Services, Office of Analysis, Nutrition and Evaluation.

Bennett, I.M., Schott, W., Krutikova, S., & Behrman, J.R. (2015). Maternal mental health, and child growth and development, in four low-income and middle-income countries. *Journal of Epidemiology and Community Health, 70*, 168-173.

Berendes, D. M., Sumner, T. A., & Brown, J. M. (2017). Safely managed sanitation for all means fecal sludge management for at least 1.8 billion people in low and middle income countries. *Environmental Science & Technology, 51*(5), 3074-3083.

Berhane, M., Yimam, H., Jibat, N., & Zewdu, M. (2018). Parents' Knowledge of Danger Signs and Health Seeking Behavior in Newborn and Young Infant Illness in Tiro Afeta District, Southwest Ethiopia: A Community-based Study. *Ethiopian Journal of Health Sciences, 28*(4).

Black, R. E., Morris, S. S., & Bryce, J. (2003). Where and why are 10 million children dying every year?. *The lancet, 361*(9376), 2226-2234.

Bloom, S. S., Wypij, D., & Gupta, M. D. (2001). Dimensions of women's autonomy and the influence on maternal health care utilization in a north Indian city. *Demography, 38*(1), 67-78.

Bogen, D. L., Hanusa, B. H., Moses-Kolko, E., & Wisner, K. L. (2010). Are maternal depression or symptom severity associated with breastfeeding intention or outcomes?. *The Journal of clinical psychiatry, 71*(8), 1069.

Bolton, P., & Tang, A. M. (2002). An alternative approach to cross-cultural function assessment. *Social psychiatry and psychiatric epidemiology, 37*(11), 537-543.

Bolton, P., Wilk, C. M., & Ndogoni, L. (2004). Assessment of depression prevalence in rural Uganda using symptom and function criteria. *Social psychiatry and psychiatric epidemiology, 39*(6), 442-447.

Bonari, L., Pinto, N., Ahn, E., Einarson, A., Steiner, M., & Koren, G. (2004). Perinatal risks of untreated depression during pregnancy. *The Canadian Journal of Psychiatry, 49*(11), 726-735.

Brickman, P., Rabinowitz, V. C., Karuza, J., Coates, D., Cohn, E., & Kidder, L. (1982). Models of helping and coping. *American psychologist, 37*(4), 368-384.

Brittain, K., Myer, L., Koen, N., Koopowitz, S., Donald, K. A., Barnett, W., ... & Stein, D. J. (2015). Risk Factors for Antenatal Depression and Associations with infant birth outcomes: results from a South African birth cohort study. *Paediatric and perinatal epidemiology, 29*(6), 505-514.

Bronte-Tinkew, J., Zaslow, M., Capps, R., Horowitz, A., & McNamara, M. (2007). Food insecurity works through depression, parenting, and infant feeding to influence overweight and health in toddlers. *The Journal of nutrition, 137*(9), 2160-2165.

Brown, J., Cairncross, S., & Ensink, J. H. (2013). Water, sanitation, hygiene and enteric infections in children. *Archives of disease in childhood, 98*(8), 629-634.

Brown, S., & Lumley, J. (2000). Physical health problems after childbirth and maternal depression at six to seven months postpartum. *BJOG: An International Journal of Obstetrics & Gynaecology, 107*(10), 1194-1201.

Bryce, J., Boschi-Pinto, C., Shibuya, K., Black, R. E., & WHO Child Health Epidemiology Reference Group. (2005). WHO estimates of the causes of death in children. *The Lancet, 365*(9465), 1147-1152.

Caliskan, D., Oncu, B., Kose, K., Ocaktan, M. E., & Ozdemir, O. (2007). Depression scores and associated factors in pregnant and non-pregnant women: A community-based study in Turkey. *Journal of Psychosomatic Obstetrics & Gynecology, 28*(4), 195-200.

Centers for Disease Control and Prevention. Depression During and After Pregnancy. (2018). Retrieved from https://www.cdc.gov/features/maternal-depression/index.html

Chatoor, I., Hirsch, R., & Persinger, M. (1997). Facilitating internal regulation of eating: A treatment model for infantile anorexia. *Infants & Young Children, 9*(4), 12-22.

Check, K. (2015). An Impact Study of Two Models of Community-Based Water Management in Uganda. *Practicing Anthropology, 37*(2), 12-16.

Chibanda, D., Mangezi, W., Tshimanga, M., Woelk, G., Rusakaniko, P., Stranix-Chibanda, L., ... & Shetty, A. K. (2010). Validation of the Edinburgh Postnatal Depression Scale among women in a high HIV prevalence area in urban Zimbabwe. *Archives of women's mental health, 13*(3), 201-206.

Child Survival Support Project, Macro International, CORE Group, MCHIP, & MCSP (2016). Knowledge, Practice and Coverage Tool. Retrieved July 23, 2020, from https://www.mcsprogram.org/resource/knowledge-practice-coverage-tool/

Choi, K. W., Sikkema, K. J., Vythilingum, B., Geerts, L., Faure, S. C., Watt, M. H., ... & Stein, D. J. (2017). Maternal childhood trauma, postpartum depression, and infant outcomes: Avoidant affective processing as a potential mechanism. *Journal of affective disorders, 211*, 107-115.

Christodoulou, J., Le Roux, K., Tomlinson, M., Le Roux, I. M., Katzen, L. S., & Rotheram-Borus, M. J. (2020). Corrigendum to" Perinatal maternal depression in rural South Africa: Child outcomes over the first two years". Journal of Affective Disorders, 247 (2019) 168-174. *Journal of affective disorders, 274*, 1223.

Chung, T. K., Lau, T. K., Yip, A. S., Chiu, H. F., & Lee, D. T. (2001). Antepartum depressive symptomatology is associated with adverse obstetric and neonatal outcomes. *Psychosomatic medicine, 63*(5), 830-834.

Chung, E. K., McCollum, K. F., Elo, I. T., Lee, H. J., & Culhane, J. F. (2004). Maternal depressive symptoms and infant health practices among low-income women. *Pediatrics, 113*(6), e523-e529.

Cohen, J. (1988). *Statistical power analysis for the behavioral sciences* (2nd ed.). New York: Psychology Press.

Cohen, S., Underwood, L. G., & Gottlieb, B. H. (Eds.). (2000). *Social support measurement and intervention: A guide for health and social scientists*. Oxford University Press.

Cooper, P. J., Murray, L., & Stein, A. (1993). Psychosocial factors associated with the early termination of breast-feeding. *Journal of Psychosomatic Research, 37*(2), 171-176.

Cooper, P. J., Tomlinson, M., Swartz, L., Woolgar, M., Murray, L., & Molteno, C. (1999). Post-partum depression and the mother-infant relationship in a South African peri-urban settlement. *The British Journal of Psychiatry, 175*(6), 554-558.

Cooper-Vince, C. E., Arachy, H., Kakuhikire, B., Vořechovská, D., Mushavi, R. C., Baguma, C., ... & Tsai, A. C. (2018). Water insecurity and gendered risk for depression in rural Uganda: A hotspot analysis. *BMC public health, 18*(1), 1143.

Costello, A. B., & Osborne, J. (2005). Best practices in exploratory factor analysis: Four recommendations for getting the most from your analysis. *Practical assessment, research, and evaluation, 10*(1), 7.

Cotrena, C., Branco, L. D., Shansis, F. M., & Fonseca, R. P. (2016). Executive function impairments in depression and bipolar disorder: association with functional impairment and quality of life. *Journal of affective disorders, 190*, 744-753.

Cuijpers, P., Weitz, E., Karyotaki, E., Garber, J., & Andersson, G. (2015). The effects of psychological treatment of maternal depression on children and parental functioning: a meta-analysis. *European Child & Adolescent Psychiatry, 24*(2), 237-245.

Cusick, S. E., & Georgieff, M. K. (2016). The role of nutrition in brain development: the golden opportunity of the "first 1000 days". *The Journal of pediatrics, 175*, 16-21.

Dambi, J. M., Corten, L., Chiwaridzo, M., Jack, H., Mlambo, T., & Jelsma, J. (2018). A systematic review of the psychometric properties of the cross-cultural translations and adaptations of the Multidimensional Perceived Social Support Scale (MSPSS). *Health and quality of life outcomes, 16*(1), 80.

Dambi, J. M., Tapera, L., Chiwaridzo, M., Tadyanemhandu, C., & Nhunzvi, C. (2017). Psychometric evaluation of the Shona version of the Multidimensional Scale of Perceived

Social Support Scale (MSPSS–Shona) in adult informal caregivers of patients with cancer in Harare, Zimbabwe. *Malawi medical journal*, *29*(2), 89-96.

Daniels, L. A., Mallan, K. M., Nicholson, J. M., Thorpe, K., Nambiar, S., Mauch, C. E., & Magarey, A. (2015). An early feeding practices intervention for obesity prevention. *Pediatrics*, *136*(1), e40-e49.

Deng A.W., Xiong R.B., Jiang T.T., Luo, Y.P., & Chen, W.Z. (2014) Prevalence and risk factors of postpartum depression in a population-based sample of women in Tangxia Community, Guangzhou. *Asian Pacific Journal of Tropical Medicine, 7*(3), 244–249.

Dennis, C. L., & McQueen, K. (2007). Does maternal postpartum depressive symptomatology influence infant feeding outcomes?. *Acta paediatrica*, *96*(4), 590-594.

De Onis, M., & Branca, F. (2016). Childhood stunting: a global perspective. *Maternal & child nutrition*, *12*, 12-26.

De Walque, D., & Kline, R. (2012). The association between remarriage and HIV infection in 13 sub-Saharan African countries. *Studies in Family Planning*, *43*(1), 1-10.

Dørheim Ho-Yen, S., Tschudi Bondevik, G., Eberhard-Gran, M., & Bjorvatn, B. (2007). Factors associated with depressive symptoms among postnatal women in Nepal. *Acta obstetricia et gynecologica Scandinavica*, *86*(3), 291-297.

Dudek, D., Jaeschke, R., Siwek, M., Maczka, G., Topor-Madry, R., & Rybakowski, J. (2014). Postpartum depression: identifying associations with bipolarity and personality traits. Preliminary results from a cross-sectional study in Poland. *Psychiatry Research, 215*(1), 69-74.

Dyson, T., & Moore, M. (1983). On kinship structure, female autonomy, and demographic behavior in India. *Population and development review*, 35-60.

Elias, C. V., Power, T. G., Beck, A. E., Goodell, L. S., Johnson, S. L., Papaioannou, M. A., & Hughes, S. O. (2016). Depressive symptoms and perceptions of child difficulty are associated with less responsive feeding behaviors in an observational study of low-income mothers. *Childhood Obesity*, *12*(6), 418-425.

Epifanio, M. S., Genna, V., De Luca, C., Roccella, M., & La Grutta, S. (2015). Paternal and maternal transition to parenthood: the risk of postpartum depression and parenting stress. *Pediatric reports*, *7*(2).

Escriba-Aguir, V. & Artazcoz, L. (2011) Gender differences in postpartum depression: A longitudinal cohort study. *Journal of Epidemiology and Community Health, 65*(4), 320–326.

Esimai, O. A., Fatoye, F. O., Quiah, A. G., Vidal, O. E., & Momoh, R. M. (2008). Antepartum anxiety and depressive symptoms: A study of Nigerian women during the three trimesters of pregnancy. *Journal of Obstetrics and Gynaecology, 28*(2), 202-203.

Ewerling, F., Lynch, J. W., Victora, C. G., van Eerdewijk, A., Tyszler, M., & Barros, A. J. (2017). The SWPER index for women's empowerment in Africa: development and validation of an index based on survey data. *The Lancet Global Health, 5*(9), e916-e923.

Familiar, I., Murray, S., Ruisenor-Escudero, H., Sikorskii, A., Nakasujja, N., Boivin, M.J., Opoka, R., & Bass, J.K. (2016). Socio-demographic correlates of depression and anxiety among female caregivers living with HIV in rural Uganda. *AIDS Care, 28*(12), 1541-1545.

Family Planning and Reproductive Health Indicators Database [Internet]. (2012). Chapel Hill (NC): MEASURE Evaluation, Carolina Population Center, University of North Carolina at Chapel Hill. Couple-years of Protection (CYP); [cited 2020 Sep 6]. Available from: http://www.cpc.unc.edu/measure/prh/rh_indicators/specific/fp/cyp.

Farías-Antúnez, S., Santos, I. S., Matijasevich, A., & de Barros, A. J. D. (2020). Maternal mood symptoms in pregnancy and postpartum depression: Association with exclusive breastfeeding in a population-based birth cohort. *Social psychiatry and psychiatric epidemiology*, 1-9.

Fatoye, F. O., Adeyemi, A. B., & Oladimeji, B. Y. (2004). Emotional distress and its correlates among Nigerian women in late pregnancy. *Journal of Obstetrics and Gynaecology, 24*(5), 504-509.

Ferrari, A. J., Charlson, F. J., Norman, R. E., Patten, S. B., Freedman, G., Murray, C. J., ... & Whiteford, H. A. (2013). Burden of depressive disorders by country, sex, age, and year: findings from the global burden of disease study 2010. *PLoS medicine, 10*(11), e1001547.

Ferrari, A. J., Somerville, A. J., Baxter, A. J., Norman, R., Patten, S. B., Vos, T., & Whiteford, H. A. (2013). Global variation in the prevalence and incidence of major depressive disorder: a systematic review of the epidemiological literature. *Psychological medicine, 43*(3), 471-481.

Field, A. (2013). *Discovering statistics using IBM SPSS statistics*. sage.

Field, S., Onah, M., van Heyningen, T., & Honikman, S. (2018). Domestic and intimate partner violence among pregnant women in a low resource setting in South Africa: a facility-based, mixed methods study. *BMC women's health, 18*(1), 119.

Fischer, M., Ramaswamy, R., Fischer-Flores, L., & Mugisha, G. (2018). Measuring and Understanding Depression in Women in Kisoro, Uganda. *Culture, Medicine, and Psychiatry*, 1-21.

Fisher, J., Mello, M. C. D., Patel, V., Rahman, A., Tran, T., Holton, S., & Holmes, W. (2012). Prevalence and determinants of common perinatal mental disorders in women in low-and lower-middle-income countries: a systematic review. *Bulletin of the World Health Organization*, *90*, 139-149.

Fisher, J. R. W., Morrow, M. M., Ngoc, N. N., & Anh, L. H. (2004). Prevalence, nature, severity and correlates of postpartum depressive symptoms in Vietnam. *BJOG: An International Journal of Obstetrics & Gynaecology*, *111*(12), 1353-1360.

Friis, H., Gomo, E., Nyazema, N., Ndhlovu, P., Krarup, H., Kæstel, P., & Michaelsen, K. F. (2004). Maternal body composition, HIV infection and other predictors of gestation length and birth size in Zimbabwe. British Journal of Nutrition, 92(5), 833-840.

Gao, L. L., Chan, S. W. C., & Mao, Q. (2009). Depression, perceived stress, and social support among first-time Chinese mothers and fathers in the postpartum period. *Research in nursing & health*, *32*(1), 50-58.

Garcia, E. R., & Yim, I. S. (2017). A systematic review of concepts related to women's empowerment in the perinatal period and their associations with perinatal depressive symptoms and premature birth. *BMC pregnancy and childbirth*, *17*(2), 347.

Garman, E. C., Schneider, M., & Lund, C. (2019). Perinatal depressive symptoms among low-income South African women at risk of depression: trajectories and predictors. *BMC pregnancy and childbirth*, *19*(1), 202.

Gausia, K., Ali, M., & Ryder, D. (2010). Diarrhoea in Bangladeshi infants and its association with postnatal depression. *Bangladesh Medical Research Council Bulletin*, *36*(1), 32-34.

Gavin, N. I., Gaynes, B. N., Lohr, K. N., Meltzer-Brody, S., Gartlehner, G., & Swinson, T. (2005). Perinatal depression: a systematic review of prevalence and incidence. *Obstetrics & Gynecology*, *106*(5), 1071-1083.

Gaynes, B. N., Gavin, N., Meltzer-Brody, S., Lohr, K. N., Swinson, T., Gartlehner, G., ... & Miller, W. C. (2005). Perinatal depression: Prevalence, screening accuracy, and screening outcomes: Summary

Gelaye, B., Rondon, M. B., Araya, R., & Williams, M. A. (2016). Epidemiology of maternal depression, risk factors, and child outcomes in low-income and middle-income countries. *The Lancet Psychiatry*, *3*(10), 973-982.

Gelaye, B., Williams, M. A., Lemma, S., Deyessa, N., Bahretibeb, Y., Shibre, T., ... & Zhou, X. H. A. (2013). Validity of the patient health questionnaire-9 for depression screening and diagnosis in East Africa. *Psychiatry research, 210*(2), 653-661.

George, C. M., Oldja, L., Biswas, S., Perin, J., Sack, R. B., Ahmed, S., ... & Bhuyian, S. I. (2016). Unsafe child feces disposal is associated with environmental enteropathy and impaired growth. *The Journal of pediatrics, 176*, 43-49.

Ghasemi, A., & Zahediasl, S. (2012). Normality tests for statistical analysis: a guide for non-statisticians. *International journal of endocrinology and metabolism, 10*(2), 486–489. https://doi.org/10.5812/ijem.3505

Glavin, K., Smith, L., & Sørum, R. (2009). Prevalence of postpartum depression in two municipalities in Norway. *Scandinavian Journal of Caring Sciences, 23*(4), 705-710.

Gorman, L. L., O'Hara, M. W., Figueiredo, B., Hayes, S., Jacquemain, F., Kammerer, M. H., ... & Sutter-Dallay, A. L. (2004). Adaptation of the structured clinical interview for DSM-IV disorders for assessing depression in women during pregnancy and post-partum across countries and cultures. *The British Journal of Psychiatry, 184*(S46), s17-s23.

Goulding, A. N., Rosenblum, K. L., Miller, A. L., Peterson, K. E., Chen, Y. P., Kaciroti, N., & Lumeng, J. C. (2014). Associations between maternal depressive symptoms and child feeding practices in a cross-sectional study of low-income mothers and their young children. *International Journal of Behavioral Nutrition and Physical Activity, 11*(1), 75.

Govindasamy, P., & Malhotra, A. (1996). Women's position and family planning in Egypt. *Studies in Family Planning*, 328-340.

Green, E. P., Blattman, C., Jamison, J., & Annan, J. (2016). Does poverty alleviation decrease depression symptoms in post-conflict settings? A cluster-randomized trial of microenterprise assistance in Northern Uganda. *Global Mental Health, 3.*

Green, E. P., Tuli, H., Kwobah, E., Menya, D., Chesire, I., & Schmidt, C. (2018). Developing and validating a perinatal depression screening tool in Kenya blending Western criteria with local idioms: A mixed methods study. Journal of affective disorders, 228, 49-59.

Grigoriadis, S., VonderPorten, E. H., Mamisashvili, L., Tomlinson, G., Dennis, C. L., Koren, G., ... & Martinovic, J. (2013). The impact of maternal depression during pregnancy on perinatal outcomes: a systematic review and meta-analysis.

Grote, V., Vik, T., von Kries, R., Luque, V., Socha, J., Verduci, E., Carlier, C., Koletzko, B., & the European Childhood Obesity Trial Study Group. (2010). Maternal postnatal depression and child growth: a European cohort study. *BMC Pediatrics, 10*(14), 1-8.

Gueron-Sela, N., Atzaba-Poria, N., Meiri, G., & Yerushalmi, B. (2011). Maternal worries about child underweight mediate and moderate the relationship between child feeding disorders and mother–child feeding interactions. *Journal of pediatric psychology, 36*(7), 827-836.

Hadley, C., Mulder, M. B., & Fitzherbert, E. (2007). Seasonal food insecurity and perceived social support in rural Tanzania. *Public health nutrition, 10*(6), 544-551.

Handiso, D. W., Ifa, Y. T., Sahiledengle, B. S., Makango, D. E., Wontamo, T. E., & Mwanri, L. M. (2020). Effect of Postpartum Depression on Exclusive Breast-Feeding Practices in Sub-Saharan Africa Countries: Systematic Review and Meta-analysis.

Hanlon, C. (2013). Maternal depression in low- and middle-income countries. *International Health, 5*(1), 4-5.

Hanlon, C., Medhin, G., Alem, A., Araya, M., Abdulahi, A., Hughes, M., ... & Prince, M. (2008). Detecting perinatal common mental disorders in Ethiopia: validation of the self-reporting questionnaire and Edinburgh Postnatal Depression Scale. *Journal of affective disorders, 108*(3), 251-262.

Harpham, T., Huttly, S., De Silva, M. J., & Abramsky, T. (2005). Maternal mental health and child nutritional status in four developing countries. *Journal of Epidemiology & Community Health, 59*(12), 1060-1064.

Harrington, W. E., Kanaan, S. B., Muehlenbachs, A., Morrison, R., Stevenson, P., Fried, M., ... & Lee Nelson, J. (2017). Maternal microchimerism predicts increased infection but decreased disease due to Plasmodium falciparum during early childhood. *The Journal of Infectious Diseases, 215*(9), 1445-1451.

Hartley, K., & Seymour, L. F. (2011, October). Towards a framework for the adoption of business intelligence in public sector organisations: the case of South Africa. In *Proceedings of the South African Institute of Computer Scientists and Information Technologists Conference on Knowledge, Innovation and Leadership in a Diverse, Multidisciplinary Environment* (pp. 116-122). ACM.

Hatløy, A., Hallund, J., Diarra, M. M., & Oshaug, A. (2000). Food variety, socioeconomic status and nutritional status in urban and rural areas in Koutiala (Mali). *Public health nutrition, 3*(1), 57-65.

Heckert, J., & Fabic, M. S. (2013). Improving data concerning women's empowerment in sub-Saharan Africa. *Studies in Family Planning, 44*(3), 319-344.

Heinig, M. J., Follett, J. R., Ishii, K. D., Kavanagh-Prochaska, K., Cohen, R., & Panchula, J. (2006). Barriers to compliance with infant-feeding recommendations among low-income women. *Journal of Human Lactation, 22*(1), 27-38.

Henderson, J. J., Evans, S. F., Straton, J. A., Priest, S. R., & Hagan, R. (2003). Impact of postnatal depression on breastfeeding duration. *Birth, 30*(3), 175-180.

Hendrick, V., Altshiler, L., Cohen, L., & Stowe, Z. (1998). Evaluation of mental health and depression during pregnancy: position paper. *Psychopharmacology Bulletin, 34*(3), 297.

Herwig, J. E., Wirtz, M., & Bengel, J. (2004). Depression, partnership, social support, and parenting: Interaction of maternal factors with behavioral problems of the child. *Journal of affective disorders, 80*(2-3), 199-208.

Hindin, M. (2012). The influence of women's early childbearing on subsequent empowerment in sub-Saharan Africa: a cross-national meta analysis. *International Center for Research on Women Fertility & Empowerment Working Paper Series, 3.*

Hoddinot, J., & Yohannes, Y. (2002). Dietary diversity as a food security indicator. FANTA. 2002. Washington DC. *Am J ClinNutr, 73.*

Howard, L. M., Oram, S., Galley, H., Trevillion, K., & Feder, G. (2013). Domestic violence and perinatal mental disorders: a systematic review and meta-analysis. *PLoS medicine, 10*(5), e1001452.

Hu, L. T., & Bentler, P. M. (1999). Cutoff criteria for fit indexes in covariance structure analysis: Conventional criteria versus new alternatives. *Structural equation modeling: a multidisciplinary journal, 6*(1), 1-55.

Huang, K. Y., Abura, G., Theise, R., & Nakigudde, J. (2017). Parental depression and associations with parenting and children's physical and mental health in a sub-Saharan African setting. *Child Psychiatry & Human Development, 48*(4), 517-527.

Hurley, K. M., Black, M. M., Papas, M. A., & Caufield, L. E. (2008). Maternal symptoms of stress, depression, and anxiety are related to nonresponsive feeding styles in a statewide sample of WIC participants. The Journal of nutrition, 138(4), 799-805.

Husain, N., Bevc, I., Husain, M., Chaudhry, I. B., Atif, N., & Rahman, A. (2006). Prevalence and social correlates of postnatal depression in a low income country. *Archives of women's mental health, 9*(4), 197-202.

Ickes, S. B., Wu, M., Mandel, M. P., & Roberts, A. C. (2018). Associations between social support, psychological well-being, decision making, empowerment, infant and young child feeding, and nutritional status in Ugandan children ages 0 to 24 months. *Maternal & child nutrition, 14*(1), e12483.

Izquierdo Alfaro, I., Olea Díaz, J., & Abad García, F. J. (2014). Exploratory factor analysis in validation studies: Uses and recommendations. *Psicothema*.

Jejeebhoy, S. J., & Sathar, Z. A. (2001). Women's autonomy in India and Pakistan: the influence of religion and region. *Population and development review*, *27*(4), 687-712.

Kabeer, N. (1998). *Money can't buy me love? Re-evaluating gender, credit and empowerment in rural Bangladesh*. Institute of Development Studies.

Kabeer, N. (1999). Resources, agency, achievements: Reflections on the measurement of women's empowerment. *Development and change*, *30*(3), 435-464.

Kabeer, N. (2001). Reflections on the measurement of women's empowerment. *Discussing Women's Empowerment: Theory and Practice*, (3).Stockholm: Swedish International Development Cooperation Agency.

Kaharuza, F. M., Bunnell, R., Moss, S., Purcell, D. W., Bikaako-Kajura, W., Wamai, N., ... & Mermin, J. (2006). Depression and CD4 cell count among persons with HIV infection in Uganda. *AIDS and Behavior*, *10*(1), 105-111.

Kaida, A., Matthews, L.T., Ashaba, S., Tsai, A.C., Kanters, S., Robak, M., Psaros, C., Kabakyenga, J., Boum, Y., Haberer, J.E., Martin, J.N., Hunt, P.W., & Bangsberg, D.R. (2014). Depression During Pregnancy and the Postpartum Among HIV-Infected Women on Antiretroviral Therapy in Uganda. *Journal of Acquired Immune Deficiency Syndromes, 67*(4), S179-S187.

Kakyo, T. A., Muliira, J. K., Mbalinda, S. N., Kizza, I. B., & Muliira, R. S. (2012). Factors associated with depressive symptoms among postpartum mothers in a rural district in Uganda. *Midwifery, 28*(3), 374-379.

Kattula, D., Sarkar, R., Sivarathinaswamy, P., Velusamy, V., Venugopal, S., Naumova, E. N., ... & Kang, G. (2014). The first 1000 days of life: prenatal and postnatal risk factors for morbidity and growth in a birth cohort in southern India. *BMJ open*, *4*(7), e005404.

Kermode, M., Herrman, H., Arole, R., White, J., Premkumar, R., & Patel, V. (2007). Empowerment of women and mental health promotion: a qualitative study in rural Maharashtra, India. *BMC public health*, *7*(1), 225.

Kerstis, B., Engström, G., Sundquist, K., Widarsson, M., & Rosenblad, A. (2012). The association between perceived relationship discord at childbirth and parental postpartum depressive symptoms: A comparisons of mothers and fathers in Sweden. *Upsala Journal of Medical Sciences, 117*(4), 430-438.

Khatun, F., Lee, T. W., Rani, E., Biswash, G., Raha, P., & Kim, S. (2018). The relationships among postpartum fatigue, depressive mood, self-care agency, and self-care action of first-time mothers in Bangladesh. *Korean Journal of Women Health Nursing, 24*(1), 49-57.

Kibaru, E. G., & Otara, A. M. (2016). Knowledge of neonatal danger signs among mothers attending well baby clinic in Nakuru Central District, Kenya: cross sectional descriptive study. *BMC research notes, 9*(1), 481.

Kijima, Y., Matsumoto, T., & Yamano, T. (2006). Nonfarm employment, agricultural shocks, and poverty dynamics: evidence from rural Uganda. *Agricultural Economics, 35*, 459-467.

Kinney, M. V., Kerber, K. J., Black, R. E., Cohen, B., Nkrumah, F., Coovadia, H., ... & Lawn, J. E. (2010). Sub-Saharan Africa's mothers, newborns, and children: where and why do they die?. *PLoS medicine, 7*(6), e1000294.

Kinyanda, E., Hoskins, S., Nakku, J., Nawaz, S., & Patel, V. (2011). Prevalence and risk factors of major depressive disorder in HIV/AIDS as seen in semi-urban Entebbe district, Uganda. *BMC psychiatry, 11*(1), 205.

Kinyanda, E., Woodburn, P., Tugumisirize, J., Kagugube, J., Ndyanabangi, S., & Patel, V. (2011). Poverty, life events and the risk for depression in Uganda. *Social psychiatry and psychiatric epidemiology, 46*(1), 35-44.

Kishor, S., & Subaiya, L. (2008). Understanding women's empowerment: a comparative analysis of Demographic and Health Surveys (DHS) data.

Kosek, M., Bern, C., & Guerrant, R. L. (2003). The global burden of diarrhoeal disease, as estimated from studies published between 1992 and 2000. *Bulletin of the world health organization, 81*, 197-204.

Kroenke, K., Spitzer, R. L., & Williams, J. B. (2001). The PHQ-9: validity of a brief depression severity measure. *Journal of general internal medicine, 16*(9), 606-613.

Kyomuhendo, G. B. (2003). Low use of rural maternity services in Uganda: impact of women's status, traditional beliefs and limited resources. *Reproductive health matters, 11*(21), 16-26.

Lambrinoudaki, I., Rizos, D., Armeni, E., Pliatsika, P., Leonardou, A., Sygelou, A., Argeitis, J., Spentzou, G., Hasiakos, D., Zervas, I., & Papadias, C. (2010). Thyroid function and postpartum mood disturbances in Greek women. *Journal of Affective Disorders, 121*(3), 278–282.

Larsson, C., Sydsjö, G., & Josefsson, A. (2004). Health, sociodemographic data, and pregnancy outcome in women with antepartum depressive symptoms. *Obstetrics & Gynecology, 104*(3), 459-466.

Lawn J, Kerber K, editors. (2006). Opportunities for Africa's Newborns: practical data, policy and programmatic support for newborn care in Africa. Cape Town: PMNCH, Save the Children, UNFPA, UNICEF, USAID, WHO.

Lee, D. T., Chan, S. S., Sahota, D. S., Yip, A. S., Tsui, M., & Chung, T. K. (2004). A prevalence study of antenatal depression among Chinese women. *Journal of Affective Disorders, 82*(1), 93-99.

Lee, L. C., Halpern, C. T., Hertz-Picciotto, I., Martin, S. L., & Suchindran, C. M. (2006). Child care and social support modify the association between maternal depressive symptoms and early childhood behaviour problems: a US national study. *Journal of Epidemiology & Community Health, 60*(4), 305-310.

Löwe, B., Spitzer, R. L., Williams, J. B., Mussell, M., Schellberg, D., & Kroenke, K. (2008). Depression, anxiety and somatization in primary care: syndrome overlap and functional impairment. *General hospital psychiatry, 30*(3), 191-199.

MacDonald, L. D., Peacock, J. L., & Anderson, H. R. (1992). Marital status: Association with social and economic circumstances, psychological state and outcomes of pregnancy. *Journal of Public Health, 14*(1), 26-34.

MacVicar, S., Berrang-Ford, L., Harper, S., Steele, V., Lwasa, S., Bambaiha, D. N., ... & IHACC Research Team. (2017). How seasonality and weather affect perinatal health: Comparing the experiences of indigenous and non-indigenous mothers in Kanungu District, Uganda. *Social Science & Medicine, 187*, 39-48.

Madlala, S. S., & Kassier, S. M. (2018). Antenatal and postpartum depression: effects on infant and young child health and feeding practices. *South African Journal of Clinical Nutrition, 31*(1), 1-7.

Mahmud, S., Shah, N. M., & Becker, S. (2012). Measurement of women's empowerment in rural Bangladesh. *World development, 40*(3), 610-619.

Makrides, M., Gibson, R. A., McPhee, A. J., Yelland, L., Quinlivan, J., & Ryan, P. (2010). Effect of DHA supplementation during pregnancy on maternal depression and neurodevelopment of young children: a randomized controlled trial. *Jama, 304*(15), 1675-1683.

Malhotra, A., & Mather, M. (1997, December). Do schooling and work empower women in developing countries? Gender and domestic decisions in Sri Lanka. In *Sociological forum* (Vol. 12, No. 4, pp. 599-630). Kluwer Academic Publishers-Plenum Publishers.

Malhotra, A., & Schuler, S. R. (2005). Women's empowerment as a variable in international development. *Measuring empowerment: Cross-disciplinary perspectives*, *1*(1), 71-88.

Manikkam, L., & Burns, J. K. (2012). Antenatal depression and its risk factors: an urban prevalence study in KwaZulu-Natal. *South African Medical Journal*, *102*(12), 940-944.

Maselko, J. (2017). Social epidemiology and global mental health: expanding the evidence from high-income to low-and middle-income countries. *Current epidemiology reports*, *4*(2), 166-173.

Mason, K. O. (1986, March). The status of women: Conceptual and methodological issues in demographic studies. In *Sociological forum* (Vol. 1, No. 2, pp. 284-300). Kluwer Academic Publishers.

Matsunaga, M. (2010). How to Factor-Analyze Your Data Right: Do's, Don'ts, and How-To's. *International journal of psychological research*, *3*(1), 97-110.

McCarter-Spaulding, D., & Horowitz, J. A. (2007). How does postpartum depression affect breastfeeding?. *MCN: The American Journal of Maternal/Child Nursing*, *32*(1), 10-17.

McCue Horwitz, S., Briggs-Gowan, M. J., Storfer-Isser, A., & Carter, A. S. (2007). Prevalence, correlates, and persistence of maternal depression. *Journal of women's health*, *16*(5), 678-691.

Mchichi Alami, K., Kadri, N., & Berrada, S. (2006). Prevalence and psychosocial correlates of depressed mood during pregnancy and after childbirth in a Moroccan sample. *Archives of women's mental health*, *9*(6), 343-346.

McKee, M. D., Zayas, L. H., & Jankowski, K. R. B. (2004). Breastfeeding intention and practice in an urban minority population: relationship to maternal depressive symptoms and mother–infant closeness. *Journal of reproductive and infant psychology*, *22*(3), 167-181.

McLearn, K. T., Minkovitz, C. S., Strobino, D. M., Marks, E., & Hou, W. (2006). The timing of maternal depressive symptoms and mothers' parenting practices with young children: implications for pediatric practice. *Pediatrics*, *118*(1), e174-e182.

McManus, B. M., & Poehlmann, J. (2012). Maternal depression and perceived social support as predictors of cognitive function trajectories during the first 3 years of life for preterm infants in Wisconsin. *Child: care, health and development*, *38*(3), 425-434.

MEASURE Evaluation Project. (2017, December 20). Family Planning and Reproductive Health Indicators Database. Retrieved July 23, 2020, from https://www.measureevaluation.org/prh/rh_indicators

Meijer, J.L., Beijers, C., van Pampus, M.G., Verbeek, T., Stolk, R.P., Milgrom, J., Bockting, C.L.H., & Burger, H. (2014). Predictive accuracy of Edinburgh Postnatal Depression Scale assessment during pregnancy for the risk of developing postpartum depressive symptoms: a prospective cohort study. *BJOG: An International Journal of Obstetrics & Gynaeocology, 121*(13), 1604-1610.

Mishra, N. K., & Tripathi, T. (2011). Conceptualising women's agency, autonomy and empowerment. *Economic and Political Weekly*, 58-65.

Mohammad, A. H., Al Sadat, N., Loh, S. Y., & Chinna, K. (2015). Validity and reliability of the hausa version of multidimensional scale of perceived social support index. *Iranian Red Crescent Medical Journal, 17*(2).

Monitoring, C. O. R. E., & Evaluation Working Group. (1999). Knowledge, practices and coverage survey. In *Knowledge, practices and coverage survey*. CORE.

Moore, S., & Croft, T. (1990). Status Report on DHS Publications and Datasets. *Population Index, 56*(2), 216-227. doi:10.2307/3644031.

Moran, V. H., Morgan, H., Rothnie, K., MacLennan, G., Stewart, F., Thomson, G., ... & Hoddinott, P. (2015). Incentives to promote breastfeeding: a systematic review. *Pediatrics, 135*(3), e687-e702.

Mubangizi, N., Kyazze, F. B., & Mukwaya, P. I. (2018). Smallholder farmers' perception and adaptation to rainfall variability in Mt. Elgon region, eastern Uganda. *International Journal of Agricultural Extension, 5*(3), 103-117.

Mugisha, J., Muyinda, H., Malamba, S., & Kinyanda, E. (2015). Major depressive disorder seven years after the conflict in northern Uganda: burden, risk factors and impact on outcomes (The Wayo-Nero Study). *BMC psychiatry, 15*(1), 48.

Muhwezi, W. W., Ågren, H., Neema, S., Koma Maganda, A., & Musisi, S. (2008). Life events associated with major depression in Ugandan primary healthcare (PHC) patients: issues of cultural specificity. *International Journal of Social Psychiatry, 54*(2), 144-163.

Mukuku, O., Mutombo, A. M., Kamona, L. K., Lubala, T. K., Mawaw, P. M., Aloni, M. N., ... & Luboya, O. N. (2019). Predictive Model for the Risk of Severe Acute Malnutrition in Children. *Journal of nutrition and metabolism, 2019*.

Murray, C. J., Lopez, A. D., & World Health Organization. (1996). The global burden of disease:

a comprehensive assessment of mortality and disability from diseases, injuries, and risk actors in 1990 and projected to 2020: summary.

Mwesiga, E. K., Mugenyi, L., Nakasujja, N., Moore, S., Kaddumukasa, M., & Sajatovic, M. (2015). Depression with pain comorbidity effect on quality of life among HIV positive patients in Uganda: a cross sectional study. *Health and quality of life outcomes, 13*(1), 206.

Nachega, J. B., Uthman, O. A., Anderson, J., Peltzer, K., Wampold, S., Cotton, M. F., ... & Mofenson, L. M. (2012). Adherence to antiretroviral therapy during and after pregnancy in low-, middle and high income countries: a systematic review and meta-analysis. *AIDS (London, England), 26*(16), 2039.

Nakasujja, N., Skolasky, R. L., Musisi, S., Allebeck, P., Robertson, K., Ronald, A., ... & Sacktor, N. (2010). Depression symptoms and cognitive function among individuals with advanced HIV infection initiating HAART in Uganda. *BMC psychiatry, 10*(1), 44.

Nakigudde, J., Musisi, S., Ehnvall, A., Airaksinen, E., & Agren, H. (2009). Adaptation of the multidimensional scale of perceived social support in a Ugandan setting. *African health sciences, 9*(2).

Nakku, J. N., Nakasi, G., & Mirembe, F. (2006). Postpartum major depression at six weeks in primary health care: prevalence and associated factors. *African health sciences, 6*(4).

Nakku, J. E. M., Rathod, S. D., Kizza, D., Breuer, E., Mutyaba, K., Baron, E. C., ... & Kigozi, F. (2016). Validity and diagnostic accuracy of the Luganda version of the 9-Item and 2-Item Patient Health Questionnaire for detecting major depressive disorder in rural Uganda. Global Mental Health, 3.

Natamba, B. K., Achan, J., Arbach, A., Oyok, T. O., Ghosh, S., Mehta, S., ... & Young, S. L. (2014). Reliability and validity of the center for epidemiologic studies-depression scale in screening for depression among HIV-infected and-uninfected pregnant women attending antenatal services in northern Uganda: a cross-sectional study. *BMC psychiatry, 14*(1), 303.

Natamba, B. K., Mehta, S., Achan, J., Stoltzfus, R. J., Griffiths, J. K., & Young, S. L. (2017). The association between food insecurity and depressive symptoms severity among pregnant women differs by social support category: a cross-sectional study. *Maternal & child nutrition, 13*(3), e12351.

Ndokera, R., & MacArthur, C. (2011). The relationship between maternal depression and adverse infant health outcomes in Zambia: a cross-sectional feasibility study. *Child: care, health and development, 37*(1), 74-81.

Ngai, F. W., & Ngu, S. F. (2015). Predictors of maternal and paternal depressive symptoms at postpartum. *Journal of psychosomatic research, 78*(2), 156-161.

Nigatu, S. G., Worku, A. G., & Dadi, A. F. (2015). Level of mother's knowledge about neonatal danger signs and associated factors in North West of Ethiopia: a community based study. *BMC research notes, 8*(1), 309.

Nolen-Hoeksema, S. (1991). Responses to depression and their effects on the duration of depressive episodes. *Journal of abnormal psychology, 100*(4), 569.

Norhayati, M. N., Hazlina, N. N., Asrenee, A. R., & Emilin, W. W. (2015). Magnitude and risk factors for postpartum symptoms: a literature review. *Journal of affective Disorders, 175*, 34-52.

O'hara, M. W., & Swain, A. M. (1996). Rates and risk of postpartum depression—a meta-analysis. *International review of psychiatry, 8*(1), 37-54.

Okeke, E. N., & Wagner, G. J. (2013). AIDS treatment and mental health: evidence from Uganda. *Social science & medicine, 92*, 27-34.

Okronipa, H. E., Marquis, G. S., Lartey, A., Brakohiapa, L., Perez-Escamilla, R., & Mazur, R. E. (2012). Postnatal depression symptoms are associated with increased diarrhea among infants of HIV-positive Ghanaian mothers. *AIDS and Behavior, 16*(8), 2216-2225.

Omoro, S. A. O., Fann, J. R., Weymuller, E. A., Macharia, I. M., & Yueh, B. (2006). Swahili translation and validation of the Patient Health Questionnaire-9 depression scale in the Kenyan head and neck cancer patient population. *The International Journal of Psychiatry in Medicine, 36*(3), 367-381.

Onyiriuka, A. N. (2006). Trends in incidence of delivery of low birth weight infants in Benin City, southern Nigeria. The Nigerian postgraduate medical journal, 13(3), 189.

Ovuga, E., Boardman, J., & Wasserman, D. (2005). The prevalence of depression in two districts of Uganda. *Social psychiatry and psychiatric epidemiology, 40*(6), 439-445.

Pao, C., Guintivano, J., Santos, H., & Meltzer-Brody, S. (2019). Postpartum depression and social support in a racially and ethnically diverse population of women. *Archives of women's mental health, 22*(1), 105-114.

Parsons, C. E., Young, K. S., Rochat, T. J., Kringelbach, M., & Stein, A. (2012). Postnatal depression and its effects on child development: a review of evidence from low-and middle-income countries. *British medical bulletin, 101*(1).

Patil, C., & Hadley, C. (2008). Symptoms of anxiety and depression and mother's marital status: An exploratory analysis of polygyny and psychosocial stress. *American Journal of Human Biology, 20*(4), 475-477.

Patil, V. H., Singh, S. N., Mishra, S., & Donavan, D. T. (2008). Efficient theory development and factor retention criteria: Abandon the 'eigenvalue greater than one' criterion. *Journal of Business Research, 61*(2), 162-170.

Pingo, J., van den Heuvel, L. L., Vythylingum, B., & Seedat, S. (2017). Probable postpartum hypomania and depression in a South African cohort. *Archives of women's mental health, 20*(3), 427-437.

Posner, K., Brent, D., Lucas, C., Gould, M., Stanley, B., Brown, G., ... & Mann, J. (2008). Columbia-suicide severity rating scale (C-SSRS). *New York, NY: Columbia University Medical Center, 10.*

Pratley, P. (2016). Associations between quantitative measures of women's empowerment and access to care and health status for mothers and their children: a systematic review of evidence from the developing world. *Social Science & Medicine, 169,* 119-131.

Preacher, K. J., & MacCallum, R. C. (2003). Repairing Tom Swift's electric factor analysis machine. *Understanding statistics: Statistical issues in psychology, education, and the social sciences, 2*(1), 13-43.

Psaros, C., Haberer, J. E., Boum, Y., Tsai, A. C., Martin, J. N., Hunt, P. W., ... & Safren, S. A. (2015). The factor structure and presentation of depression among HIV-positive adults in Uganda. *AIDS and Behavior, 19*(1), 27-33.

Rahman, A., Bunn, J., Lovel, H., & Creed, F. (2007). Maternal depression increases infant risk of diarrhoeal illness:–a cohort study. Archives of disease in childhood, 92(1), 24-28.

Ramchandani, P., & Psychogiou, L. (2009). Paternal psychiatric disorders and children's psychosocial development. *The Lancet, 374*(9690), 646-653.

Ramsay, M., Gisel, E. G., McCusker, J., PhD, F. B., & PhD, R. P. (2002). Infant sucking ability, non-organic failure to thrive, maternal characteristics, and feeding practices: a prospective cohort study. *Developmental Medicine & Child Neurology, 44*(6), 405-414.

Reid, K. M., & Taylor, M. G. (2015). Social support, stress, and maternal postpartum depression: A comparison of supportive relationships. *Social Science Research, 54,* 246-262.

Roberts, B., Ocaka, K. F., Browne, J., Oyok, T., & Sondorp, E. (2008). Factors associated with post-traumatic stress disorder and depression amongst internally displaced persons in northern Uganda. *BMC psychiatry*, *8*(1), 38.

Robertson, R. C., Manges, A. R., Finlay, B. B., & Prendergast, A. J. (2019). The human microbiome and child growth–first 1000 days and beyond. *Trends in microbiology*, *27*(2), 131-147.

Rochat, T. J., Richter, L. M., Doll, H. A., Buthelezi, N. P., Tomkins, A., & Stein, A. (2006). Depression among pregnant rural South African women undergoing HIV testing. *Jama*, *295*(12), 1373-1378.

Roomruangwong, C., Kanchanatawan, B., Sirivichayakul, S., & Maes, M. (2016). Antenatal depression and hematocrit levels as predictors of postpartum depression and anxiety symptoms. *Psychiatry research*, *238*, 211-217.

Salk, R. H., Hyde, J. S., & Abramson, L. Y. (2017). Gender differences in depression in representative national samples: Meta-analyses of diagnoses and symptoms. *Psychological Bulletin*, *143*(8), 783.

Sandberg, J., Pettersson, K. O., Asp, G., Kabakyenga, J., & Agardh, A. (2014). Inadequate knowledge of neonatal danger signs among recently delivered women in southwestern rural Uganda: a community survey. *PLoS One*, *9*(5), e97253.

Sarkar, N., Bardaji, A., Peeters Grietens, K., Bunders-Aelen, J., Baingana, F., & Criel, B. (2018). The social nature of perceived illness representations of perinatal depression in rural Uganda. *International journal of environmental research and public health*, *15*(6), 1197.

Sawyer, A., Ayers, S., & Smith, H. (2010). Pre-and postnatal psychological wellbeing in Africa: a systematic review. *Journal of affective disorders*, *123*(1-3), 17-29.

Schatz, E., & Williams, J. (2012). Measuring gender and reproductive health in Africa using demographic and health surveys: the need for mixed-methods research. *Culture, health & sexuality*, *14*(7), 811-826.

Schlaudecker, E. P., Steinhoff, M. C., & Moore, S. R. (2011). Interactions of diarrhea, pneumonia, and malnutrition in childhood: recent evidence from developing countries. *Current opinion in infectious diseases*, *24*(5), 496.

Schwarzenberg, S. J., & Georgieff, M. K. (2018). Advocacy for improving nutrition in the first 1000 days to support childhood development and adult health. *Pediatrics*, *141*(2), e20173716.

Sen, A. (1985). Well-being, agency and freedom: The Dewey lectures 1984. *The journal of philosophy*, *82*(4), 169-221.

Shain, R. N., Piper, J. M., Newton, E. R., Perdue, S. T., Ramos, R., Champion, J. D., & Guerra, F. A. (1999). A randomized, controlled trial of a behavioral intervention to prevent sexually transmitted disease among minority women. *New England Journal of Medicine*, *340*(2), 93-100.

Shidhaye, P., & Giri, P. (2014). Maternal Depression: A Hidden Burden in Developing Countries. *Annals of Medical and Health Sciences Research*, *4*(4), 463–465. http://doi.org/10.4103/2141-9248.139268

Singer, L. T., Davillier, M., Preuss, L., Szekely, L., Hawkins, S., Yamashita, T., & Baley, J. (1996). Feeding interactions in infants with very low birth weight and bronchopulmonary dysplasia. *Journal of developmental and behavioral pediatrics: JDBP*, *17*(2), 69.

Singla, D. R., Kumbakumba, E., & Aboud, F. E. (2015). Effects of a parenting intervention to address maternal psychological wellbeing and child development and growth in rural Uganda: a community-based, cluster-randomised trial. *The Lancet Global Health*, *3*(8), e458-e469.

Smedberg, J., Lupattelli, A., Mårdby, A. C., Øverland, S., & Nordeng, H. (2015). The relationship between maternal depression and smoking cessation during pregnancy—a cross-sectional study of pregnant women from 15 European countries. *Archives of women's mental health*, *18*(1), 73-84.

Solar, O., & Irwin, A. (2010). A conceptual framework for action on the social determinants of health.

Stein, A., Lehtonen, A., Harvey, A. G., Nicol-Harper, R., & Craske, M. (2009). The influence of postnatal psychiatric disorder on child development. *Psychopathology*, *42*(1), 11-21.

Stellenberg, E. L., & Abrahams, J. M. (2015). Prevalence of and factors influencing postnatal depression in a rural community in South Africa. *African journal of primary health care & family medicine*, *7*(1), 1-8.

Stewart, R. C. (2007). Maternal depression and infant growth–a review of recent evidence. *Maternal & child nutrition*, *3*(2), 94-107.

Stewart, D. E., Robertson, E., Dennis, C. L., Grace, S. L., & Wallington, T. (2003). Postpartum depression: Literature review of risk factors and interventions. *Toronto: University Health Network Women's Health Program for Toronto Public Health*.

Stewart, R. C., Umar, E., Tomenson, B., & Creed, F. (2014). Validation of the multi-dimensional scale of perceived social support (MSPSS) and the relationship between social support, intimate partner violence and antenatal depression in Malawi. *BMC psychiatry*, *14*(1), 180.

Suri, R., Altshuler, L., Hellemann, G., Burt, V. K., Aquino, A., & Mintz, J. (2007). Effects of antenatal depression and antidepressant treatment on gestational age at birth and risk of preterm birth. *American Journal of Psychiatry*, *164*(8), 1206-1213.

Surkan, P. J., Kennedy, C. E., Hurley, K. M., & Black, M. M. (2011). Maternal depression and early childhood growth in developing countries: systematic review and meta-analysis. *Bulletin of the World Health Organization*, *89*, 607-615.

Surkan, P. J., Patel, S. A., & Rahman, A. (2016). Preventing infant and child morbidity and mortality due to maternal depression. *Best practice & research Clinical obstetrics & gynaecology*, *36*, 156-168.

Swindale, A., & Bilinsky, P. (2006). Development of a universally applicable household food insecurity measurement tool: process, current status, and outstanding issues. *The Journal of nutrition*, *136*(5), 1449S-1452S.

Tannous, L., Gigante, L. P., Fuchs, S. C., & Busnello, E. D. (2008). Postnatal depression in Southern Brazil: prevalence and its demographic and socioeconomic determinants. *BMC psychiatry*, *8*(1), 1.

Tatone-Tokuda, F., Dubois, L., & Girard, M. (2009). Psychosocial determinants of the early introduction of complementary foods. *Health Education & Behavior*, *36*(2), 302-320.

Thompson, B., & Daniel, L. G. (1996). Factor analytic evidence for the construct validity of scores: A historical overview and some guidelines.

Tol, W. A., Ebrecht, B., Aiyo, R., Murray, S. M., Nguyen, A. J., Kohrt, B. A., ... & Nakku, J. (2018). Maternal mental health priorities, help-seeking behaviors, and resources in post-conflict settings: a qualitative study in eastern Uganda. *BMC psychiatry*, *18*(1), 39.

Tomlinson, M., Cooper, P. J., Stein, A., Swartz, L., & Molteno, C. (2006). Post-partum depression and infant growth in a South African peri-urban settlement. *Child: care, health and development*, *32*(1), 81-86.

Tsai, A. C., Bangsberg, D. R., Emenyonu, N., Senkungu, J. K., Martin, J. N., & Weiser, S. D. (2011). The social context of food insecurity among persons living with HIV/AIDS in rural Uganda. *Social science & medicine*, *73*(12), 1717-1724.

Tsai, A. C., Bangsberg, D. R., Frongillo, E. A., Hunt, P. W., Muzoora, C., Martin, J. N., & Weiser, S. D. (2012). Food insecurity, depression and the modifying role of social support among people living with HIV/AIDS in rural Uganda. *Social science & medicine, 74*(12).

Tumwine, J. K., Thompson, J., Katua-Katua, M., Mujwajuzi, M., Johnstone, N., Wood, E., & Porras, I. (2002). Diarrhoea and effects of different water sources, sanitation and hygiene behaviour in East Africa. *Tropical Medicine & International Health, 7*(9), 750-756.

Tumwine, J., Thompson, J., Katui-Katua, M., Mujwahuzi, M., Johnstone, N., & Porras, I. (2003). Sanitation and hygiene in urban and rural households in East Africa. *International journal of environmental health research, 13*(2), 107-115.

Turney, K. (2013). Perceived instrumental support and children's health across the early life course. *Social Science & Medicine, 95*, 34-42.

Uganda Bureau of Statistics. (2017). ICF. The Uganda Demographics and Health Survey 2016: Key Indicators Report.

Ugandan Ministry of Finance, Planning and Economic Development, International Monetary Fund. (2003).Uganda poverty status report, 2003: achievements and pointers for the PEAP revision. Washington, DC.

Ugandan Ministry of Health (2012). Uganda AIDS indicator survey (UAIS). Kampala, Uganda: government of Uganda, Ministry of Health.

Underwood, L., Waldie, K., D'Souza, S., Peterson, E. R., & Morton, S. (2016). A review of longitudinal studies on antenatal and postnatal depression. *Archives of Women's Mental Health, 19*(5), 711-720.

Upadhyay, U. D., Gipson, J. D., Withers, M., Lewis, S., Ciaraldi, E. J., Fraser, A., ... & Prata, N. (2014). Women's empowerment and fertility: a review of the literature. *Social Science & Medicine, 115*, 111-120.

Upadhyay, U. D., & Karasek, D. (2010). Women's Empowerment and Achievement of Desired Fertility in Sub-Saharan Africa. *International Perspectives on Sexual and Reproductive Health, 38*(2), 78-89.

Upadhyay, U. D., & Karasek, D. (2012). Women's empowerment and ideal family size: an examination of DHS empowerment measures in Sub-Saharan Africa. *International perspectives on sexual and reproductive health*, 78-89.

Vaezi, A., Soojoodi, F., Banihashemi, A. T., & Nojomi, M. (2019). The association between social support and postpartum depression in women: A cross sectional study. *Women and Birth, 32*(2), e238-e242.

Vaivada, T., Akseer, N., Akseer, S., Somaskandan, A., Stefopulos, M., & Bhutta, Z. A. (2020). Stunting in Childhood: an overview of global burden, trends, determinants, and drivers of decline. *The American journal of clinical nutrition, 112*(Supplement_2), 777S-791S.

Verkuijl, N. E., Richter, L., Norris, S. A., Stein, A., Avan, B., & Ramchandani, P. G. (2014). Postnatal depressive symptoms and child psychological development at 10 years: a prospective study of longitudinal data from the South African Birth to Twenty cohort. *The Lancet Psychiatry, 1*(6), 454-460.

Vesga-Lopez, O., Blanco, C., Keyes, K., Olfson, M., Grant, B. F., & Hasin, D. S. (2008). Psychiatric disorders in pregnant and postpartum women in the United States. *Archives of general psychiatry, 65*(7), 805-815.

Victora, C. G., Horta, B. L., De Mola, C. L., Quevedo, L., Pinheiro, R. T., Gigante, D. P., ... & Barros, F. C. (2015). Association between breastfeeding and intelligence, educational attainment, and income at 30 years of age: a prospective birth cohort study from Brazil. *The lancet global health, 3*(4), e199-e205.

Villegas, L., McKay, K., Dennis, C. L., & Ross, L. E. (2011). Postpartum depression among rural women from developed and developing countries: a systematic review. The Journal of Rural Health, 27(3), 278-288.

Wagner, G. J., Ghosh-Dastidar, B., Dickens, A., Nakasujja, N., Okello, E., Luyirika, E., & Musisi, S. (2012). Depression and its relationship to work status and income among HIV clients in Uganda. *World Journal of AIDS, 2*(3), 126.

Wagner, G. J., Ghosh-Dastidar, B., Robinson, E., Ngo, V. K., Glick, P., Musisi, S., & Akena, D. (2017). Effects of depression alleviation on work productivity and income among HIV patients in Uganda. *International journal of behavioral medicine, 24*(4), 628-633.

Wagner, G. J., Holloway, I., Ghosh-Dastidar, B., Kityo, C., & Mugyenyi, P. (2011). Understanding the influence of depression on self-efficacy, work status and condom use among HIV clients in Uganda. *Journal of psychosomatic Research, 70*(5), 440-448.

Wagner, G. J., Ngo, V., Glick, P., Obuku, E. A., Musisi, S., & Akena, D. (2014). Integration of DEPression Treatment into HIV Care in Uganda (INDEPTH-Uganda): study protocol for a randomized controlled trial. *Trials, 15*(1), 248.

Wang, Y., Moe, C. L., Null, C., Raj, S. J., Baker, K. K., Robb, K. A., ... & Armah, G. (2017). Multipathway quantitative assessment of exposure to fecal contamination for young children in low-income urban environments in Accra, Ghana: the SaniPath analytical approach. *The American journal of tropical medicine and hygiene, 97*(4), 1009-1019.

Waqas, A., Elhady, M., Dila, K. S., Kaboub, F., Nhien, C. H., Al-Husseini, M. J., ... & Huy, N. T. (2018). Association between maternal depression and risk of infant diarrhea: a systematic review and meta-analysis. *Public health, 159*, 78-88.

Weiser, S. D., Tsai, A. C., Gupta, R., Frongillo, E. A., Kawuma, A., Senkungu, J., ... & Bangsberg, D. R. (2012). Food insecurity is associated with morbidity and patterns of healthcare utilization among HIV-infected individuals in a resource-poor setting. *AIDS (London, England), 26*(1), 67.

Wemakor, A., & Iddrisu, H. (2018). Maternal depression does not affect complementary feeding indicators or stunting status of young children (6–23 months) in Northern Ghana. *BMC research notes, 11*(1), 408.

Wemakor, A., & Mensah, K. A. (2016). Association between maternal depression and child stunting in Northern Ghana: a cross-sectional study. *BMC public health, 16*(1), 869.

Weobong, B., Akpalu, B., Doku, V., Owusu-Agyei, S., Hurt, L., Kirkwood, B., & Prince, M. (2009). The comparative validity of screening scales for postnatal common mental disorder in Kintampo, Ghana. *Journal of affective disorders, 113*(1-2), 109-117.

Weobong, B., Soremekun, S., Ten Asbroek, A. H., Amenga-Etego, S., Danso, S., Owusu-Agyei, S., ... & Kirkwood, B. R. (2014). Prevalence and determinants of antenatal depression among pregnant women in a predominantly rural population in Ghana: The DON population-based study. *Journal of affective disorders, 165*, 1-7.

Weobong, B., ten Asbroek, A. H., Soremekun, S., Gram, L., Amenga-Etego, S., Danso, S., ... & Kirkwood, B. R. (2015). Association between probable postnatal depression and increased infant mortality and morbidity: findings from the DON population-based cohort study in rural Ghana. *BMJ open, 5*(8).

Will, J. C., Khavjou, O., Finkelstein, E. A., Loo, R. K., & Gregory-Mercado, K. Y. (2007). One-year changes in glucose and heart disease risk factors among participants in the WISEWOMAN programme. *European Diabetes Nursing, 4*(2), 57-63.

Wisner, K. L., Bogen, D. L., Sit, D., McShea, M., Hughes, C., Rizzo, D., ... & Wisniewski, S. W. (2013). Does fetal exposure to SSRIs or maternal depression impact infant growth?. *American Journal of Psychiatry, 170*(5), 485-493.

Wittkowski, A., Gardner, P. L., Bunton, P., & Edge, D. (2014). Culturally determined risk factors for postnatal depression in Sub-Saharan Africa: a mixed method systematic review. *Journal of affective disorders, 163*, 115-124.

Woldetensay, Y. K., Belachew, T., Ghoph, S., Kantelhardt, E. J., Biesalski, H. K., & Scherbaum, V. (2019). The Effect of Maternal Depressive Symptoms on Infant Feeding Practices in Rural Ethiopia: Community Based Birth Cohort Study.

Wolf, A. W., De Andraca, I., & Lozoff, B. (2002). Maternal depression in three Latin American samples. *Social Psychiatry and Psychiatric Epidemiology, 37*(4), 169-176.

Wolf, K., & Frese, M. (2018). Why husbands matter: Review of spousal influence on women entrepreneurship in sub-Saharan Africa. *Africa Journal of Management, 4*(1), 1-32.

Woody, C. A., Ferrari, A. J., Siskind, D. J., Whiteford, H. A., & Harris, M. G. (2017). A systematic review and meta-regression of the prevalence and incidence of perinatal depression. *Journal of affective disorders, 219*, 86-92.

Woolhouse, H., Gartland, D., Perlen, S., Donath, S., & Brown, S. J. (2014). Physical health after childbirth and maternal depression in the first 12 months post-partum: results of an Australian nulliparous pregnancy cohort study. *Midwifery, 30*(3), 378-384.

World Health Organization. (2003). Infant and young child feeding: a tool for assessing national practices, policies and programmes.

World Health Organization. (2008). Maternal mental health and child health and development in low and middle income countries: report of the meeting, Geneva, Switzerland, 30 January-1 February, 2008.

World Health Organization. (2009). WHO child growth standards and the identification of severe acute malnutrition in infants and children: joint statement by the World Health Organization and the United Nations Children's Fund.

World Health Organization. (2010). UNAIDS: Global Report: UNAIDS report on the global AIDS epidemic. *Geneva: WHO.*

World Health Organization. (2011). The global burden of disease: 2004 update. 2008. 51. Larsson C, Sydsjo G, Josefsson A. Health, sociodemographic data, and pregnancy outcome in women with antepartum depressive symptoms. Obstetrics and Gynecology, 2004, 104:459-466.

World Health Organization. (2019). World malaria report 2019. World Health Organization. https://apps.who.int/iris/handle/10665/330011.

Wortman, C. B. (1984). Social support and the cancer patient: Conceptual and methodologic issues. *Cancer, 53*, 2339-2360.

Wu, M., Li, X., Feng, B., Wu, H., Qiu, C., & Zhang, W. (2014). Poor sleep quality of third-trimester pregnancy is a risk factor for postpartum depression. *Medical science monitor: international medical journal of experimental and clinical research, 20,* 2740.

Yağmur, Y., & Ulukoca, N. (2010). Social support and postpartum depression in low-socioeconomic level postpartum women in Eastern Turkey. *International journal of public health, 55*(6), 543-549.

Yuan, K. H., & Bentler, P. M. (1998). Structural equation modeling with robust covariances. *Sociological methodology, 28*(1), 363-396.

Zaers, S., Waschke, M., & Ehlert, U. (2008). Depressive symptoms and symptoms of post-traumatic stress disorder in women after childbirth. *Journal of Psychosomatic Obstetrics & Gyneocology, 29*(1), 61-71.

Zakama, A. K., Ozarslan, N., & Gaw, S. L. (2020). Placental Malaria. *Current Tropical Medicine Reports,* 1-10.

Zimet, G. D., Dahlem, N. W., Zimet, S. G., & Farley, G. K. (1988). The multidimensional scale of perceived social support. *Journal of personality assessment, 52*(1), 30-41.

MODIFIED PATIENT HEALTH QUESTIONNAIRE-9

	Over the past week, how often have you been bothered by any of the following problems? [PHQ-9]	
1	Little interest or pleasure in doing things	- 0 days (Not at all) - 1 - 3 days (Several days) - 4 - 5 days (More than half days) - 6 – 7 days (Nearly every day)
2	Feeling down, depressed or hopeless	(Same as above)
3	Trouble falling asleep, staying asleep, or sleeping too much	(Same as above)
4	Feeling tired or having little energy	(Same as above)
5	Poor appetite or overeating	(Same as above)
6	Feeling bad about yourself – or that you're a failure or have let yourself or your family down	(Same as above)
7	Trouble concentrating on things, such as [reading the newspaper or watching television]	(Same as above)
8	Moving or speaking so slowly that other people could have noticed. Or , the opposite – being so fidgety or restless that you have been moving around a lot more than usual.	(Same as above)
9	Thoughts that you would be better off dead or of hurting yourself in some way	(Same as above)
10	*(If the person mentioned any problems above)* How difficult have those problems made it for you to do your work, take care of things at home, or get along with other people?	- Not difficult at all - Somewhat difficult - Very difficult - Extremely difficult

MODIFIED MULTIDIMENSIONAL SCALE OF PERCEIVED SOCIAL SUPPORT

For each belief below, ask the person if the AGREE or DISAGREE with the statement. If they Agree, ask, "Do you Agree a little or Agree a lot?" If they Disagree, ask, "Do you Disagree a little or Disagree a lot?" Mark only one response for each belief.				
Belief	**Disagree a Lot**	**Disagree a Little**	**Agree a little**	**Agree a lot**
42. There is a special person who is around when I am in need.	1	2	3	4
43. There is a special person with whom I can share joys and sorrows.	1	2	3	4
44. My family really tries to help me.	1	2	3	4
45. I get the emotional help & support I need from my family.	1	2	3	4
46. I have a special person who is a real source of comfort to me.	1	2	3	4
47. My friends really try to help me.	1	2	3	4
48. I can count on my friends when things go wrong.	1	2	3	4
49. I can talk about my problems with my family.	1	2	3	4
50. I have friends with whom I can share my joys and sorrows.	1	2	3	4
51. There is a special person in my life who cares about my feelings.	1	2	3	4
52. My family is willing to help me make decisions.	1	2	3	4
53. I can talk about my problems with my friends.	1	2	3	4
Multidimensional Scale of Perceived Social Support Score: Add response to questions #42-53 and divide by 12. *Significant Other Subscale*: Add 42, 43, 46, and 51 and divide by 4. *Family Subscale*: Sum 44, 45, 49 and 52 and divide by 4. *Friends subscale*: Sum 47, 48, 50, and 53 and divide by 4	_____ points